Practical Priorities for
FIBROMYALGIA
Recovery

12 Simple Strategies for Creating a
Chemical-Free Life, Revving Up Your Immune
System, and Improving Your Symptoms

KATHY K. NORMAN
WITH VICTOR D. NORMAN, M.D.

Practical Priorities for Fibromyalgia Recovery: 12 Simple Strategies for Creating a Chemical-Free Life, Revving Up Your Immune System, and Improving Your Symptoms

Any internet addresses or company or product information printed in this book are offered as a resource and are not intended in any way to be or to imply an indorsement by the authors, Kathy K. Norman or Victor D. Norman. Nor do the authors vouch for the existence, content, or services of these sites beyond the use as resources for the reader. This book does not replace the advice of a medical professional. Consult your physician before making any changes to your diet, medications, lifestyle, normal activities, or regular health plan.

Scripture taken from the Holy Bible, NEW INTERNATIONALVERSION®, NIV® Copyright © 1973, 1978, 1984, 2011 by Biblica, Inc.® Used by permission. All rights reserved worldwide.

ISBN 978-0-578-82208-2

Published by Kathy K. Norman

Praise for Practical Priorities for Fibromyalgia Recovery

"Don't just take Kathy Norman's word for it, listen to her doctor husband, Victor Norman MD, too. Practical Priorities for Fibromyalgia Recovery: 12 Simple Strategies for Creating a Chemical-Free Life, Revving Up Your Immune System, and Improving Your Symptoms takes the reader on Kathy's journey to fibromyalgia recovery and shares Vic's explanation of why her advice is medically sound. Most impressively, their common-sense suggestions for change can be easily followed by taking small steps and adapting their advice to fit your own needs. I observed Kathy in the early stages of her recovery when she changed her diet with a simple rule, "Eat nothing from a box," and saw how the change to eating real food began to relieve some of her pain. As this book explains, achieving significant relief requires changes in numerous areas of exposure to harmful chemicals, such as personal hygiene products and types of household cleaners. Anyone with an inflammatory illness or chronic pain who is willing to try these simple changes will be well on their way to better health."

William H. Coleman M.D. Ph.D., past-president American Academy of Family Medicine

"Kathy Norman and her physician husband, Dr. Victor D. Norman, have written an extraordinary guide: *Practical Priorities for Fibromyalgia Recovery: 12 Simple Strategies for Creating a Chemical-Free Life, Revving Up Your Immune System, and Improving Your Symptoms*. Kathy begins with her personal story about how she struggled with the debilitating disease fibromyalgia, and step by step throughout the book, she and her husband describe the simple change of lifestyle that brought her healing and relief from constant pain. I highly recommend this eye-opening book because it will change your life in wonderful ways! I don't have fibromyalgia, but the information is so useful for everyone, I plan to reread this guide numerous times, using it as a constant reference to take charge of my health and home, giving copies to my friends, and practicing its well-documented advice."

Denise George, author, and founder of Writers for Life

"In this timely book, Kathy and Vic Norman have made a significant contribution to the understanding of fibromyalgia and how to address it. Kathy's testimonial of her personal struggles dealing with fibromyalgia and eventually coping with the disease through lifestyle changes is a compelling read, well written, and clearly elaborated. Vic, a family physician and medical educator, provides helpful comments following each of Kathy's chapters. Fibromyalgia sufferers and their loved ones will find *Practical Priorities for Fibromyalgia Recovery: 12 Simple Strategies for Creating a Chemical-Free Life, Revving Up Your Immune System, and Improving Your Symptoms* a must read. Anyone who merely wants a healthier lifestyle will appreciate the encouraging narrative, helpful tips, and nutritious recipes. In addition, counselors, chaplains, pastors, and medical clinicians will discover a valuable resource from Kathy's and Vic's insights through the years of pain and emotional stress Kathy experienced before finding a way to *improved health and activity. Personally, I found Kathy's narrative and suggestions brimming with hope and inspiration, and Vic's medical observations a reassuring anchor in my own attempts to develop a healthier and more fulfilling lifestyle."*

M. Dennis Herman, D. Min., retired pastor, chaplain, and missionary colleague of the Normans at the Clínica Bautista, Barranquilla, Colombia

"After 25 years of battling fibromyalgia, buying numerous books, and trying all kinds of medications, I finally found what I was looking for in Kathy Norman's book, written with her physician husband, Dr. Victor D. Norman. Practical Priorities for Fibromyalgia Recovery: 12 Simple Strategies for Creating a Chemical-Free Life, Revving Up Your Immune System, and Improving Your Symptoms gave me simple strategies to make healthy lifestyle changes. I knew I needed to overhaul everything, but I thought I didn't have the time or motivation to try. I knew I needed an uncomplicated approach to an anti-inflammatory diet, but I wasn't prepared to take chemicals out of my life because it seemed like more than I had the energy to do. Kathy made that much easier than I had anticipated. The practical priority strategies were easy to incorporate into my life with the step-by-step approach presented in the book. Prior to following the steps in the book, I was in constant pain. Any movement was difficult. After several months of slowly removing most chemicals from my home and monitoring my food intake to make sure I left out processed food and ate real food, I was a completely different person. My body responded by allowing me to resume normal functions without severe pain. This book changed my life. I wholeheartedly recommend it."

Kay M. Williams, MA, LMFT, psychotherapist specializing in first responder trauma, beta reader and beta tester for Practical Priorities for Fibromyalgia Recovery

Dedication

This book is dedicated to all the fabulous fierce fibro fighters. Living with fibromyalgia is not for the faint of heart. You are phenomenal warriors battling insidious chronic illness with determination and grace. I see you going to work, raising children, completing chores, running errands, and rising up to face the day while constantly struggling with excruciating pain and debilitating fatigue. I feel the darkness of despair this daunting disease creates in even the most optimistic of souls. I hear your voices clamoring for a glimmer of hope that one day your symptoms will improve. Fibromyalgia is an invisible illness. But you are not invisible. Not to me.

Contents

Dedication ix

Introduction. xiii

Priority 1: Understand Fibromyalgia 1

Priority 2: Find Your Focus 15

Priority 3: Deal with Depression. .25

Priority 4: Identify Your Support Network. 35

Priority 5: Recognize We Live in a Toxic World. 47

Priority 6: Remove Scented Products from Your Home 55

Priority 7: Exchange Harmful Household Products for
    Safer Ones. 63

Priority 8: Eliminate Most Processed Food from Your Diet.75

Priority 9: Make Smart Real Food Choices 87

Priority 10: Move Every Day 105

Priority 11: Get Enough Sleep 117

Priority 12: Analyze Your Unique Results. 129

Appendix I Recipes for Nontoxic Cleaners and Household
    Products 143

Appendix II Real Food Recipes 153

Appendix III Resources for Further Reading 205

Acknowledgments. 211

About the Authors. 213

Endnotes 215

Introduction

DO YOU WANT to breeze through each day brimming with health and vitality? That sounds like either an awesome goal or a commercial for a new super vitamin. For me, it was just a nebulous idea floating around the outer edges of my real life. I felt well most of the time and, besides, I was too busy to give much thought to creating a healthy lifestyle. Adulting was time-consuming and the years raced by in a flash while I was teaching school, birthing babies, scrubbing countertops, ministering in Colombia, writing devotionals, overloading at church, working at the office, cooking, chauffeuring children, paying bills, and juggling a hundred other responsibilities.

Along the way, I made the occasional stab at ramping up my health status. I tried diet programs (not to get healthier but to lose enough weight to fit back into my favorite pair of jeans), joined an exercise group (not because I valued aerobics but because a bunch of friends were participating), and took afternoon walks around my subdivision (because I liked fresh air and enjoyed chatting with the neighbors). If I was occasionally sick, I had the ultimate resource close at hand. My husband is a doctor! Vic could prescribe something to treat whatever bug was going around that month or refer me to a specialist when I needed a consult. As soon as I recovered from each temporary illness, I returned to my routine life and remained oblivious to the long-term health effects of my shortsighted viewpoint.

Our bodies are designed to be whole and well, but I never thought about making intentional choices to stay healthy. We are equipped with a remarkable immune system to fend off germs and disease. I had access to a bountiful supply of fruits, vegetables, grains, nuts, and seeds to keep my immune system functioning at optimal capacity. But I didn't care. I ate whatever I wanted. Household products and personal grooming items are filled with potentially harmful substances. Yet, I mindlessly spritzed cleaners and slathered on cosmetics without pausing to consider the toxic ingredients used to manufacture them.

I still would be completely apathetic and woefully uninformed about the overwhelming toxicity that bombards us every single day if I hadn't been diagnosed with fibromyalgia, a chronic illness that has no definitive cause or cure.

Fibromyalgia turned my world upside down. Before the diagnosis, I was vibrant, active, energetic, and enthusiastic about life. Afterward, I was racked with horrible pain, debilitating fatigue, and crushing despair.

When I lost my health, I lost my innate sense of self and my understanding of who I was meant to be in the world. I struggled to hold on to my faith, which for more than half a century had been my anchor and rock. Day after day of unremitting pain and debilitating fatigue left me feeling doomed, weak, hopeless, and questioning God. I was a wreck.

I wasted an entire year feeling sorry for myself before I got so sick and tired of being sick and tired that I decided to quit complaining and take action. I embarked on a personal research project looking for ways to improve my fibromyalgia symptoms and create a healthier life. I clicked my way through reams of data in cyberspace searching for ideas.

I'm not some nerdy expert with a lab coat and five advanced degrees. If you're looking for piles of footnoted information, statistical analysis, and indecipherable scientific jargon, keep browsing through the healthy living section at the bookstore. There's bound to be a meticulously researched academic book in there somewhere. On the other hand, if you want to know how an ordinary woman contracted an incurable chronic illness, learned to cope with the fallout, and eventually recovered, read on.

As I searched for ways to deal with my fibromyalgia dilemma, I discovered that we live in a shockingly toxic world that adversely affects our health. It was mind boggling how many harmful things lurked in my pantry, fridge, cupboards, and cosmetic drawer. I eventually created specific simple strategies for coping with my illness by decreasing my exposure to toxic substances and increasing my openness to making healthy lifestyle changes.

I didn't have to go it alone during this learning process. My husband, Vic, is a retired family physician and medical educator. His medical knowledge was an invaluable asset as I looked for ways to improve my health. Vic drops by in each chapter to share a physician's perspective on the practical priorities presented in the book.

Every doctor I consulted, including Vic, told me there was no definitive cure for fibromyalgia. I was too stubborn to let that teensy fact weaken my resolve to find something that might help me cope with the debilitating symptoms. My research methods were quite haphazard. I roamed around cyberspace like a deranged disease detective looking for clues.

Now that I'm writing this book, I wish I had kept scrupulous notes on every article I read, who said this and that, where I gleaned each nugget of information. But at the time, I wasn't thinking about writing a book. I was focused solely on finding a way to improve my horrible symptoms. I'll share with you how I did it, what I learned, the lifestyle changes I made, and the unanticipated results. For readers who want additional information on the discoveries I made, I'll include citations throughout the book that you can peruse in the endnotes.

I stumbled upon my first big clue when I read about the suspected link between exposure to harmful chemicals in processed foods and household products I used every day and the onset of fibromyalgia, as well as a myriad of other chronic illnesses, including many autoimmune diseases, diabetes, allergies, asthma, cardiovascular disease, and some types of cancer.

I explored ways to minimize the impact of these harmful substances. It quickly became apparent that creating a chemical-free existence would require me to change almost everything about the way I did life. Vic and I decided early on that there were two nonnegotiable criteria for each lifestyle change I made.

- **Do no harm.** One of the most well-known promises new doctors make when they take the Hippocratic Oath is, "First, do no harm." This became our mantra. Whatever I tried had to be safe. I certainly didn't want to make things worse than they already were.
- **Be practical.** I didn't have the energy nor the inclination to implement changes that were convoluted and complicated. Whatever I tried had to be realistic and relatively simple.

At first, I found a lot of weird suggestions both for coping with chronic illness and for creating a healthier life. Some of the ideas sounded flaky (wearing a copper bracelet or a necklace made of crystals), some sounded dangerous (stopping all medications prescribed by my doctor), and some suggestions sounded so complicated that I felt defeated before I even started (making strange juice concoctions from obscure fruits and roots not likely to be found at my local Big Star or Piggly Wiggly grocery stores). I needed a more sensible plan.

My first goal was to learn as much as I could about my specific illness. People with fibromyalgia have a broad array of symptoms in multiple parts of the body. The most universal symptom is debilitating pain in multiple joints and muscles. It's the symptom that wreaked the most havoc on my ability to function normally. I was determined to find a way to reduce my excruciating pain.

Over the course of a year, I developed simple strategies for coping with fibromyalgia and creating a healthier life. Even though the strategies were simple, implementing them was a challenge. I had to change almost everything in my daily routine: the way I cook, what I eat, how I clean, and the type of cosmetics and personal care items I use. It was a tremendous amount of work.

If I had known at the beginning how much I would ultimately have to redesign my life, I might never have started. However, since I discovered random facts here and there over time, I was able to modify my routine little by little. Because this was a slow process of discovery, I never felt overwhelmed. I will share detailed information about every aspect of the plan I created and suggest ways to implement change in small increments so that you won't feel overwhelmed either.

I will help you understand the dynamics of your illness, the specific foods and household products that are harmful, how to detoxify your life, how to boost your immune system to optimize health, and show you practical ways to integrate change into your daily routine.

I'm honored to share my story with you. I know that my story will not be the same as yours. Each one of us is unique. And that's a good thing. It would be an awfully boring world if we were all alike.

What is your story? Are you sick? Do you have fibromyalgia? Have you been diagnosed with some other chronic illness? Are you currently healthy but want to do whatever you can to prevent illness? Are you interested in designing a chemical-free life? Do you want to improve your immune system? Are you looking for ways to create a healthier life for yourself and your family?

In this book, I'll share my story and give you tools to rewrite yours. Vic will drop by to give you a doctor's viewpoint. It's up to you to decide what to do with this information. Your choices will be impacted by your personality, your family dynamics, your worldview, and your current health status. No matter what your goals are, this book can help you write a new and healthier story.

At the end of each chapter, I'll recommend three specific steps for you to take. You can choose when and how to implement the changes you choose to make. Every positive step you take will move you that much closer to creating a healthier reality.

If you are not currently sick, that is wonderful. The information shared in this book can help you stay that way and give you tools for preventing the onset of chronic illness in the future.

If you are one of the millions of people in the world who have fibromyalgia or some other type of chronic illness, I want to share some words of hope. You can get better. There are different degrees of debilitation in the disease process. Maybe you have been chronically ill for twenty years. Perhaps you just got a fibromyalgia diagnosis last month. Maybe you feel okay most of the time but have some really bad days at other times. Perhaps you feel horrible every second of every day.

I don't know how sick you are. I can't promise that you will get well and never be sick again. I was so decimated by pain and despair I was skeptical that anything could improve my particular symptom pattern. However, I was unwilling to resign myself to a lifetime of illness without at least trying to find a way to improve.

There are different degrees of healing. Maybe this book will help you learn to manage your symptoms better. Perhaps you will find some ideas in these pages for coping with chronic illness. Maybe some of the things shared here will help you have more good days than bad days. It will be an adventure to see where the journey takes you.

One thing is certain. If you do nothing, you will stay exactly where you are. But if you make the changes suggested in these pages, you can improve your symptoms and create a healthier life. You may even completely recover. That may sound too good to be true. I wouldn't believe it myself in a million years except for this: it happened to me.

Practical Priorities for FIBROMYALGIA Recovery

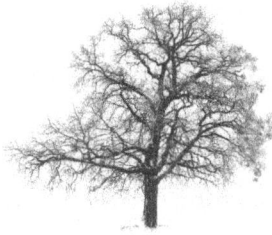

Priority 1: Understand Fibromyalgia

TWO DAYS BEFORE I almost died, I zoomed around as usual trying to cram as much as possible into my day off. I washed five loads of laundry, ironed all of our scrub suits for the coming week, baked several batches of festive cookies, did some last-minute Christmas shopping, and got the guest rooms ready for out-of-town family coming to spend the holidays at our house.

On Monday morning, December 21, 2009, I jumped out of bed, threw on my scrubs, and headed to work. I stopped by the grocery store, bank, and pharmacy on the way to the office. At 9:00 a.m. I hurried to my desk, put on my headphones, and booted up the computer to transcribe the medical notes Vic had dictated over the weekend. I enjoyed working in my husband's family practice clinic. In addition to medical transcription, I made appointments, worked on charts, filed lab reports, wrote letters, answered the phone, and translated for our Spanish-speaking patients. Life was *muy bien*. But it wouldn't stay that way for long.

The last morning patient headed out the door and the office staff headed out to lunch at a nearby restaurant that had a nice quick buffet. I was slightly skittish about going there because I'm allergic to shellfish and the buffet choices included shrimp and crab. Since I had never had a problem eating there before, I shrugged off the nagging worry and filled my plate.

My chicken, rice, and vegetables smelled wonderful. I grabbed my fork and swallowed the first delicious bite. Within two minutes I knew something was terribly wrong. My lips, face, tongue, and throat began to swell. I had difficulty breathing. My chest felt like an elephant was standing on it. I was going into anaphylactic shock. It had happened before when I had come into accidental contact with shellfish. My lungs were shutting down. I grabbed my purse and rummaged around for the EpiPen and Benadryl that I keep with me at all times. The allergic reaction was so severe that Vic decided we should go straight to the emergency room since we were only five minutes away from the hospital.

He hustled me out to the car and we raced to the ER. As soon as we arrived, an IV line was inserted into my vein and I was given an injection of epinephrine while the ER staff monitored my vital signs. The swelling in my throat rapidly worsened. I had tremendous difficulty breathing. I was given another injection of epinephrine with no result. My airway was still constricted. If my throat completely closed and my stats continued to deteriorate, I could die from anaphylactic shock. After a third injection, Vic and the ER physician were discussing hooking me up to a ventilator when the symptoms finally started to abate. I stayed in the emergency room several hours for observation and was sent home when the danger had passed.

Soon after this frightening experience, we closed the office for the Christmas holidays. My mother, children, and grandchildren arrived at our home to stay with us for a week. I felt horrible the whole time they were there but muddled through the festivities with a fake smile plastered on my face. The first week of January the office reopened and I dragged myself back to work. I was incredibly tired and extremely weak. I barely had the energy to make it through the day. I thought my body was just having trouble recovering from the stress of the severe anaphylactic reaction, all the epinephrine I was given in the emergency room, and the hectic holiday season.

The end of January I developed some puzzling new symptoms of numbness in my face, arms, and legs, and severe muscle and joint pain all over my body. I had a medical checkup including laboratory analysis. All of the test results returned within normal limits.

Vic suspected that I had developed fibromyalgia with a strong chronic fatigue component. He had several patients with fibromyalgia who had a similar symptom pattern. The onset of fibromyalgia often follows some type of trauma like the severe anaphylactic reaction I had experienced. A formal diagnosis could not be made until the symptoms had persisted for at least three to six months and I was evaluated by a specialist. But the signs were all there. I became a statistic. I joined the ranks of the millions of people in our country who have fibromyalgia.

I'd love to tell you how smart and proactive I was about immediately taking charge of my illness and aggressively investigating ways to improve my symptoms. That would be an inspiring story. But it would be a lie.

The truth is, after I was diagnosed with fibromyalgia, I wasted a year struggling with pain, fatigue, and feeling sorry for myself. I tried to remain optimistic. I woke up every morning hoping I would finally feel better. Instead, I woke up every morning feeling worse than I had the day before.

I cut back on my hours at work, resigned from a volunteer position at church, and tried to get as much rest as possible. Nothing helped. I was morphing from an active woman fully engaged in life into a stay-at-home invalid and I hated it. I didn't feel like going to many social events so I attended my own self-pity parties.

An entire year passed. The holidays rolled around again. New Year's Day 2011 came and went. I woke up on a bleak January morning and struggled to get out of bed. I managed to brush my teeth, comb my hair, and shuffle to the den where I plopped down on the couch, wrapped myself in a warm blanket, and settled in with my Bible, my prayer list, and the laptop.

I read a psalm or two and a chapter from the book of John. Then I prayed for friends and family. I scarcely knew what to pray for myself. All of the doctors I saw told me fibromyalgia was lifelong and incurable. What was I supposed to pray for exactly?

In the quietness of that cold morning I stared out the windows at the trees behind my house. They all looked as dead as I felt. I love the woodsy landscape surrounding our home. I enjoy watching the trees change through the seasons of the year. Even in winter they are weirdly beautiful with twisted trunks and bare branches splayed against the gray sky.

I thought about how the trees would look when spring came again. Leaves would bud and unfurl on all of those empty branches until every limb of every tree was full and green and dancing with the wind.

In the stillness of that moment, a tiny thought bubbled to the surface of my consciousness. Maybe I was like those trees: seemingly lifeless at the moment but holding the promise of renewal somewhere down deep inside. Something had triggered this disease in me. Maybe something could turn it off.

I'm not a research scientist nor a medical professional. I had no idea how or where to start looking for ways to feel better. I shifted on the couch and my hand grazed the laptop resting on the cushion beside me. As I absentmindedly stroked the shiny black surface, it occurred to me that I had access to an almost unlimited supply of information literally at my fingertips. There might be something in the reams of data streaming through cyberspace that could help me. I powered up the laptop and started to search for clues.

I scoured the internet to find out everything I could about my specific illness. I discovered that I wasn't alone. According to the National Fibromyalgia Association, ten million people in the United States have fibromyalgia. It is estimated that 3-6% of the population around the world has the disease.[1] The number varies depending on who you ask, but any way you parse it, millions of people struggle to cope with fibromyalgia.

I ran across all manner of fibromyalgia factoids. It's a multi-systemic disease that affects patients of all ages and backgrounds. Symptoms vary from patient to patient. Common symptoms include severe pain in muscles and joints, chronic fatigue, difficulty concentrating, insomnia, headaches, irritable bowel syndrome, nausea, sensitivity to temperature changes, numbness, anxiety, and depression. And that's just a few of them. I found one list that named over 200 symptoms![2]

Although folks with fibromyalgia have different symptom patterns, they also have some similarities. Over the years he treated fibromyalgia patients in his private medical practice, Vic noticed they had some things in common.

- They seem to have some type of genetic predisposition for developing fibromyalgia. There are many cases of multiple members of the same family having the disease, which suggests there is some kind of genetic flaw.
- They show signs of a weakened immune system such as having recurrent infections like sinusitis or being susceptible to viral illnesses.
- They have been diagnosed with one or more other chronic illnesses prior to the onset of fibromyalgia.
- They have a prior history of multiple allergies.
- They experience mild to severe depression, either as a separate disease or as an ancillary symptom to fibromyalgia.
- They suffer from an inability to concentrate, often referred to as fibro fog, that results in disorganization and confusion.

- They have a lifelong history of exposure to toxic substances in processed food, cleaning products, cosmetics, pesticides, and other household products.
- They experience some type of severe physical, mental, emotional, or spiritual trauma prior to the onset of the disease.

It was eerie how accurately I fit this pattern. I had other chronic illnesses, multiple allergies, was dealing with severe depression for the first time in my life, experienced the trauma of a major allergic reaction prior to diagnosis, had been exposed to toxic substances for decades, and apparently had a flawed immune system. I couldn't do anything about some of the things on the list. I couldn't change my genetic makeup, my past exposure to toxic substances, or my previous medical history. But I could focus on how to deal with depression and fibro fog, search for ways to rev up my immune system, and look for practical ways to decrease my exposure to toxic chemicals.

I didn't have the slightest idea where this would lead. However, I felt a hazy aura of hope hovering around the keyboard as I searched for possibilities. Whatever I discovered might help me find ways to cope with and, perhaps, even improve my symptoms. I went for it.

Dr. Norman Drops By

I watched my wife, Kathy, as her health steadily deteriorated after she was diagnosed with fibromyalgia. It was frustrating that I had no quick solution to mitigate her increasing symptoms. I was there every step of the way as she investigated ways to cope with fibromyalgia. We discussed every possibility she discovered in her online research. In each chapter, I'll share my medical perspective on the strategies Kathy created to deal with chronic illness.

I am a Board-Certified Family Physician. I have practiced medicine for over 30 years; first as a missionary doctor in Colombia, South America, and then in my private medical office in the friendly little town of Red Bay, Alabama. After I retired from private practice, I was a medical educator affiliated with the teaching faculty of the School of Medicine at the University of Alabama.

During the course of my medical career, I focused on preventing disease as well as treating acute illnesses. If you are currently fairly healthy, the information we share in this book can help you stay that way by showing you how to rev up your immune system and giving you the tools you need to create a chemical-free life to maximize the possibility of preventing the onset of disease as you age.

If you currently suffer from fibromyalgia or another chronic illness, implementing the strategies in this book can help improve your symptoms and increase your chances for healing.

If you have been diagnosed with any illness, it is important to have the information you need to help you deal with the symptom pattern. A wide spectrum of factors is involved in the disease process for every illness. Because this book is geared primarily toward people who have been diagnosed with fibromyalgia, it is important to understand this particular disease process.

Fibromyalgia symptoms often ebb and flow. If you have fibromyalgia, it is quite common to feel somewhat better for a few days and then experience a sudden flare-up that makes you feel much worse. Because of this pattern, many patients with fibromyalgia often wait a significant amount of time before seeing a physician for their symptoms. The mindset that, "I'll feel better tomorrow," is very common. I saw patients who had symptoms for several weeks, months, or even years before seeking medical attention.

Fibromyalgia symptoms are usually widespread throughout the entire body. Patients with fibromyalgia have symptoms in various systems in the body. The disease affects the musculo-skeletal system which includes muscles, joints, and tendons around the joints. It commonly affects the nervous system and the immune system. It may also cause symptoms in the gastro-intestinal, endocrine, neurological, and genitourinary systems.

Fibromyalgia can be difficult to diagnose because the symp-toms are multisystemic and often vague. The symptoms don't necessarily follow a set pattern. In other diseases, there is a set of symptoms that are typical. For example, cough, fever, shortness of breath, and sputum production commonly indicate the presence of pneumonia. The diagnosis can be confirmed by x-raying the lungs. Treatment is fairly straightforward: antibi-otics, oxygen, respiratory treatments, and hospital admission if the pneumonia is particularly severe.

In fibromyalgia the symptoms don't add up. There is no universally accepted cause for fibromyalgia. Physicians dis-agree on how to even classify this illness. Because fibromyalgia causes pain in muscles and joints, it was initially thought to be an inflammatory illness related to arthritis. Some researchers argue it should be classified solely as a neurological disorder that affects the nervous system. Other researchers think that some type of autoimmune system dysfunction is involved. They note that some autoimmune diseases have symptom patterns quite similar to fibromyalgia and that fibromyalgia patients often have one or more autoimmune diseases in addition to fibromyalgia. Decades of treating patients who suffer from fibromyalgia plus my daily personal observation of Kathy during her illness, indi-cate to me that the autoimmune system is intricately involved in fibromyalgia. I believe that researchers will eventually discover atypical autoimmune activity in patients who have this disease. It is little wonder the disease is so difficult to treat when doctors can't even agree on something as basic as a cause or a classifi-cation for fibromyalgia.

There is no definitive test to diagnose fibromyalgia. The diagnosis is made using a diagnosis of exclusion in which the doctor eliminates every other possible cause for the symptoms. There are no clear-cut treatments for fibromyalgia. There are a number of drugs used to attempt to moderate the pain the disease causes, but their track record is neither clear nor strong.

Many doctors feel uncomfortable with having no diagnostic test and no definitive treatment. Physicians have been trained to make a diagnosis, treat the disease, and help the patient. Some are uneasy admitting, "I don't know what to do." Because fibromyalgia is difficult to diagnose, some doctors ignore the patient's complaints or discount the symptoms.

If you have a fibromyalgia symptom pattern, you need to consult a doctor who listens with concern to the medical history you relate, takes the time necessary to ascertain what is wrong, evaluates your symptoms, and does what he can to help you cope with your disease. If your current doctor is not adequately addressing your fibromyalgia issues, you need to consider finding another physician who will.

Fibromyalgia patients exhibit varying symptom patterns but they have one thing in common. Most patients experience some type of significant trauma prior to the onset of the disease. Precipitating traumatic events usually fall under one of the following five scenarios:

The patient has an acute illness.
The acute illness may be a viral illness or some type of infection such as the flu, a severe urinary tract infection, strep throat, pneumonia, or another acute illness. Normally, these types of illnesses run their course in a few days to a few weeks. But sometimes the symptoms linger, the patient never recovers, often gets worse, and is eventually diagnosed with fibromyalgia.

The patient has a severe allergic reaction.
I believe this was a precipitating factor in the onset of fibromyalgia in Kathy's particular case. She had a severe anaphylactic reaction to shellfish. There are many types of allergens. Common allergens include fragrance, chemicals, latex, food additives, insect stings and bites, and various foods such as shellfish, milk, soy, gluten, and peanuts. Allergic reactions can range from the relatively mild response of a small itching bump on the skin to the extremely severe response of anaphylaxis which causes respiratory distress and can lead to death.

The patient experiences some type of physical trauma.
Being severely injured in a motor vehicle accident is a good example of physical trauma. The patient does not improve from the accident injuries as expected. The patient continues to have lingering symptoms. The inflammation caused by the injuries in the motor vehicle accident may be a factor in precipitating the onset of fibromyalgia symptoms.

The patient experiences a severe emotional trauma.
Examples of emotional trauma include experiencing grief and loss after the death of a loved one, going through a messy divorce, discovering your child is addicted to drugs, being the sole caregiver for an aging parent, or spiraling into depression after a particularly traumatic relational event. Depression is a normal short-term response to emotional trauma. Depression that lasts for longer than six months is considered pathological. For example, it is normal to be depressed for approximately six months after someone close to you dies. A patient may continue to grieve for much longer than that, even years. However, after six months the patient should at least be at the point of starting to show some gradual improvement. Severe depression that lasts for longer than six months needs to be evaluated by a physician.

Some patients are misdiagnosed as having lingering situational depression after experiencing grief and loss, when actually the symptoms indicate the onset of fibromyalgia.

The patient experiences some type of spiritual trauma.

This type of trauma may be more difficult to evaluate. There are many factors involved including the patient's particular religious background, how important her faith is in her daily life, and her perception of how she should relate to God and to other people. Spiritual questions may arise when a relationship is broken, a patient feels wounded by conflict within her church, or a tragic event occurs that causes the patient to question her faith and to question God. If the patient is unable to work through the spiritual trauma, it can precipitate a full-blown fibromyalgia onset.

Any form of trauma can cause an inflammatory response, as well as affect the immune system. If you have fibromyalgia, it is likely that you experienced one or more of these five types of trauma prior to diagnosis.

Understanding as much as you can about your disease, including possible precipitating factors, lays a good foundation for creating strategies to improve your symptoms.

Your Turn

At the end of each chapter, I will suggest three practical activities to help you process the information we share in small manageable increments. These will include completing specific tasks, making lists, and answering questions to help you focus your thoughts. I encourage you to record your responses, either directly in the book, or in a separate journal. Check off activities as you do them. Complete the steps at your own pace as you design a personalized plan for coping with chronic illness that fits your unique lifestyle.

1. I had a very specific reason for wanting to get healthier. I was looking for a way to decrease my fibromyalgia symptoms. One of my main priorities was to create a chemical-free life. This book is designed to help people who have fibromyalgia. However, creating a chemical-free life is useful for anyone interested in healthy living. Exposure to toxic chemicals has been linked to the onset of a wide variety of illnesses including many types of cancer and a broad spectrum of chronic autoimmune diseases. Why would you like to get healthier? Why would you like to create a chemical-free lifestyle? Do you have fibromyalgia or another chronic illness? Do you want to boost your immune system? Prevent disease? Create a healthier home environment for your family? What is your current story?

2. If you have fibromyalgia, did you experience one of the five types of life trauma described in this chapter? Which one(s) happened to you prior to the onset of your chronic illness?

3. What is your current symptom pattern? Put a checkmark by each symptom that you currently have. In the first date/scale column, write today's date and rate the severity of each symptom you list on a scale of one to ten with ten being the highest level of severity. For example, if you have occasional mild nausea you might choose to rate that a one. If you have constant excruciating pain in multiple joints, that might be a ten. If you have headaches that occur once every week or so you might rate that particular symptom as a five. This list will give you a tangible picture of your current symptom pattern. You will look at the list again later in the book.

My Symptoms   **Date/Rate 1-10**   **Date/Rate 1-10**

___Anxiety
___Bladder discomfort
___Concentration difficulty
___Constipation
___Depression
___Diarrhea
___Dizziness
___Fatigue
___Food intolerance
___Headaches
___Insomnia
___Irritable bowel syndrome
___Light sensitivity
___Memory difficulty
___Mental fog
___Migraines
___Nausea
___Numbness
___Pain in joints
___Pain in muscles
___Sleep disruption
___Sound sensitivity
___Tingling in hands and feet
___Temperature sensitivity
___Touch sensitivity
___Other

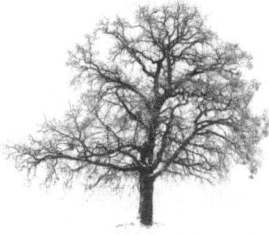

Priority 2: Find Your Focus

FIBROMYALGIA LEFT ME unfocused and disorganized. This was weirdly atypical for me. I'm usually a meticulous planner. In fact, I'm so into orchestrating life, I've been accused of dictatorial behavior on more than one occasion. (I don't understand this misguided attitude. I obviously know the right way to do whatever it is that needs doing. Why can't my family and friends just accept this and get with the program?)

My organizational skills evaporated into a cloud of fibro fog and daily debilitation. I was a muddled mess. I didn't have a spreadsheet, calendar of daily objectives, or any kind of structured plan to implement my personal research project. Chronic illness robbed me of the capacity to plan a methodical approach to solving my current dilemma. How was I going to find ways to improve my symptoms?

My brain was fuzzy but fortunately my fingers were still working (for the most part). I sat on the couch with the laptop perched on my knees, fired up the search engine, and typed whatever keyword wandered into my head that day. I tried fibromyalgia, chronic illness, healthy living, coping, pain, fatigue, trauma, life stinks. (Well, maybe not that last one; but, it's how I felt.)

Due to some inexplicable quirk in cyberspace, most of my initial searches led to links of a bunch of famous people hawking fitness products, exercise equipment, and weight loss programs. Okay, so my shape is more fluffy than svelte, but I wasn't looking for a weight loss program or a fitness plan. I was looking for ways to decrease my fibromyalgia symptoms. I just wanted the pain and fatigue to go away.

After weeks of frustration and dead ends, I finally stumbled onto an article that immediately captured my attention. I don't know how in the world I ended up there. You know how it is: click, click, click – and suddenly, without meaning to, you are binge watching Stephen Colbert riff on the last three weeks of political shenanigans. But I digress.

I inadvertently clicked my way to a link that described the suspected relationship between sensitivity to the chemicals in scented products and chronic illness. The article described how scented products are made from a variety of synthetic toxic ingredients including harmful volatile organic compounds (VOCs). VOCs was the first of many new chemical words and phrases I eventually added to my vocabulary.

I don't remember the name of the article or the author or anything about that site except that something huge clicked for me as I read that piece. I felt like a ridiculously happy cartoon character with the light bulb of epiphany perched over my head. I was intrigued because of my past medical history.

I have multiple allergies including extreme sensitivity to perfume and other scented products. Allergies are based on an abnormal response in the immune system. While fibromyalgia is not currently classified as an autoimmune disease, some physicians think abnormalities in the immune system are linked to the onset of fibromyalgia. Some autoimmune diseases, such as lupus, have symptom patterns strikingly similar to fibromyalgia. Some folks with fibromyalgia have other chronic illnesses that are classified as autoimmune diseases. Was some type of dysfunction in my immune system responsible, at least in part, for my symptom pattern? Was it possible that there was a connection between exposure to chemicals used in scents and fibromyalgia? Fragrance is not the only chemical added to products during the manufacturing process. There are a lot of chemicals in a lot of products. Could there be other harmful chemicals that contributed to my current unhealthy state? If I found out what they were and eliminated them from my home, could I improve my fibromyalgia symptoms and create a healthier reality? Even at this early stage in my research, it was obvious that I would need to find ways to move toward a chemical-free life. That was going to require making a lot of changes in the way I did almost everything.

My mindset was the first thing I had to change. Every doctor I had seen said there was no cure for fibromyalgia. Everything I had read, so far, indicated that this diagnosis was a lifelong sentence so I might as well get used to it. I was focused solely on the horrible reality that I was doomed to wake up every single day with severe pain, chronic fatigue, and an ever-increasing cascade of awful symptoms. If I was going to stay sick the rest of my life no matter what I did, why bother making any lifestyle changes? I might as well accept my fate, curl up on the couch, and watch television all day (assuming I possessed sufficient energy to flip channels on the remote).

And if you had said to me while I was stuck in that frame of mind, "Hmmm. I don't think that attitude will be particularly helpful in reaching your goal to feel better," I would have replied, "Too bad. It is what it is. So, there! If you don't like it, you can just go take a flying leap off the nearest cliff. Preferably landing in a moat. Full of alligators. And swamp rats. And maybe a few hungry piranhas."

I was a tiny bit miffed and perhaps a teensy bit sensitive from constant pain and feeling wretched every single day. The truth is, I desperately needed to change my focus to have any hope at all of changing my current pitiful health status.

That is easier said than done. After a year of constant pain and illness, I was convinced this was my new normal and I was positive there was nothing I could do to change that fact. I was negative and bitter. I had forgotten how to be thankful for anything. And worst of all, my normally exuberant faith in God was shredded into tatters.

It's strange that this particular illness compromised my faith to such a degree. I had experienced the negative side of life before. I had been dismissed by folks I thought were friends. I had been disappointed by church people and church leaders. I had other chronic illnesses. People I loved had died. I knew first hand that bad things happen to good people all the time. In the past, whatever circumstances came my way, I had confronted them head on with my faith intact.

Not now. I questioned the very idea of a God who cared about humanity in general, and me in particular. Oh, I still prayed every now and then. But my prayers were not filled with hope and faith. They were more along the line of, "Dear God. I hate being sick. And if you exist, I hate you." Am I a stellar example of a woman of faith or what?

Anger about why God would allow this level of pain to consume my life was a legitimate initial response to being so sick; but it was not a place that I could stay. My belief in God had been my core touchstone for over five decades. I wanted to find my way back to hope and faith.

There have been many attempts to explain what faith means based on verses in the Bible like this one: "Now faith is being sure of what we hope for and certain of what we do not see." (Hebrews 11:1 NIV)

That sounds more like a riddle than a clarification. We can dissect that verse, read it in the original Greek, discuss it in somber theological overtones, and make it fit our preconceived notion of what faith should be. The truth is that faith means different things to different people.

People all over the globe have been diagnosed with fibromy-algia. Readers of this book may be from many different cultures, countries, ethnicities, religious traditions, and denominational affiliations. Your beliefs may not be the same as mine. Perhaps you consider yourself to be spiritual but not religious. Maybe you don't think of yourself as either one. We each have our own ideas about what the word *faith* means.

My personal definition of faith is based on what I believe about God. This belief informs how I see the world and how I relate to other people. My faith can be succinctly summed up in one small sentence that contains one big idea. God loves us and he wants us to love him back and love other people.

Maybe faith in God is not a major touchstone in your life at all. You may find your center in a different place than I find mine. Your touchstone may be family, friends, yoga, meditation, nature, pets, books, or quiet spaces. Your faith may be in God, spiritual practices, medicine, or yourself. Perhaps, you feel at peace when you are hiking in the mountains or watching the sun set over the ocean. Maybe your faith is strengthened by being with other believers in a particular church congregation. Wherever your faith resides, it is quite common for that faith to be compromised by chronic illness. To most effectively cope with disease and summon the courage to create a healthier way forward, it is essential to get in touch with the place that feeds your soul.

The method used to hold on to faith in times of great distress varies from person to person. We are unique individuals. It is natural that we will have unique responses to faith issues. It is important to find and hold on to your personal touchstones as you consider ways to improve your physical symptoms.

I rehabilitated my fractured faith by focusing on four things.
- I practiced honest prayer. I told God the truth when I prayed. "I'm mad. I don't trust you. You will have to help me find my way back to faith. I can't do this alone." If God

is all-knowing, then he knew what I was thinking anyway so I might as well admit my true feelings. Honest prayer was my pathway to honest response and restoration.

- I remembered God's activity in my life in the past. I had experienced love and blessings. An abundance of good things and good people had come my way before. It was within the realm of probability that good things could come my way again.

- I practiced intentional gratitude. Every day I expressed thanks for something in my life. I had a roof over my head, clean water, food, the necessities of existence, family, friends, and the possibility of improving my health. Making gratitude lists for what I still had took my focus off of what I had lost to chronic illness.

- I acknowledged that finding my way back to faith would take time. It did. During the course of my personal research project, my faith ebbed and flowed. (Hope note: I eventually got there.)

While I focused on reconnecting with my faith, I also worked on changing my negative mindset about my current physical limitations. I was sick with what I had been told was an incurable chronic illness. I knew I needed to change my focus from obsessing about the problem to looking for possible ways to improve. I determined I would make any lifestyle changes that held even minimal hope of helping me.

I had a stare down contest with reality. My habits were deeply ingrained by the time I was diagnosed with fibromyalgia. Almost every one of my daily habits involved exposure to some type of potentially toxic chemical. I was accustomed to eating things from boxes and bags. I had used certain household products and personal care items for my entire adult life. I was emotionally invested in my habitual way of doing things. Change might be hard but staying sick the rest of my life would be harder. Unwillingness to change is a crippling state of mind. Openness to new ideas and new ways of doing things became a liberating opportunity for me to become a healthier woman.

My lifelong proclivity for organization eventually kicked back in. I love lists. I wrote down three initial goals for searching for ways to improve my symptoms.

- I would make only those lifestyle changes that were practical and could do no harm.
- I would focus on positive possibilities and hang on to my touchstone of faith.
- I would search for information about harmful chemicals in things I used every day and find ways to create a chemical-free life.

Looking at my written list was a visible reminder of my commitment to find a way to cope with fibromyalgia. I changed my mindset from problems to possibilities, began the process to reconnect with my faith touchstone, and listed concrete goals for my research project. I found my focus and held on to the hope that it would change my reality.

Dr. Norman Drops By

If you are ready to tackle your fibromyalgia symptoms, you need to focus on the positive possibilities for improvement and commit to taking concrete steps to move toward creating a healthier life. I recommend you begin by doing two things:

- Schedule an appointment with your family physician for a complete checkup and laboratory analysis.
- Learn all you can about your disease.

Doctors normally wait for three to six months to diagnose fibromyalgia. If symptoms have been present for less than six months, the usual protocol is for the physician to do a clinical evaluation that includes laboratory analysis to see if there could be some other cause for the symptoms.

There are other diseases that mimic the symptoms of fibromyalgia. These include, but are not limited to, lupus, rheumatoid arthritis, anemia, Parkinson's disease, Sjogren's syndrome, and multiple sclerosis.

There are other less serious conditions that may also mimic fibromyalgia which take time to diagnose and treat. For example, a patient with mononucleosis may present with symptoms of pain and fatigue. There are laboratory tests that can be done to determine if a patient has mononucleosis. It can take up to six months for mononucleosis symptoms to resolve. There are other viruses that have no objective tests for diagnosis that also can cause a person to be sick for up to six months before they start to recover. Thyroid disorders may show a symptom pattern similar to fibromyalgia. Laboratory readings may be within normal limits at first. After the onset of thyroid illness, it can take three to six months for abnormal thyroid levels to show up in laboratory analysis.

Although there are no specific tests designed to diagnose fibromyalgia, there are ancillary problems that sometimes go along with fibromyalgia that can be diagnosed with appropriate laboratory work. You need evaluation to make sure that you do not have a thyroid or vitamin deficiency, anemia, elevated rheumatoid factor, or other complicating issue. Your physician can write orders for you to have any needed laboratory analysis. The basic evaluation should include the following:

- Complete metabolic profile (CMP)
- Complete blood count (CBC)
- Thyroid panel
- Vitamin D level
- Vitamin B 12 level
- Rheumatoid factor and ANA

Your physician may recommend other laboratory tests. You need to have some or all of these tests repeated each year. Your first series of laboratory tests at the time of the onset of your symptoms may be within normal limits. However, one or two years later when the laboratory tests are repeated at your annual checkup, it is not uncommon for the results to show new findings such as a Vitamin D deficiency, a low B 12 level, a thyroid problem, or other abnormalities that were not present when you were first diagnosed. These conditions can be treated with medications. For example, if you have vitamin deficiencies, your condition may improve greatly by taking the appropriate vitamin supplements.

I know that when you are ill, it can be frustrating to wait for a diagnosis. However, it is important to be patient if your doctor tells you that there may be a delay in confirming your diagnosis. Your physician can treat your illness only when a correct diagnosis is made. A doctor does not want to treat someone for fibromyalgia if another illness is responsible for the symptoms.

Kathy started her investigation into possible causes and help for fibromyalgia by reading everything she could find about this specific disease and about chronic illness in general. It is important for patients with any type of illness to gather information to help them understand their particular disease.

As a family physician, I found providing patient education to be an invaluable resource. On every office visit, I spent time helping each patient understand his or her illness. I explained the disease, discussed the causes of the disease, and gave the patient information concerning what to expect during the course of that particular disease process. I described the possible treatment options, what I considered the best option for that particular patient, and any possible side effects connected with the treatment.

The amount of education I could give each patient was limited by the time I had to spend with him or her before moving on to the next appointment. Therefore, I also provided written materials about the illness for the patient to take home. I gave patients pamphlets and information sheets, and loaned books to them from the small library I kept at my office.

I also suggested that patients use reliable online resources such as:

- Medline Plus https://www.nlm.nih.gov/medlineplus
- The Centers for Disease Control and Prevention http://www.cdc.gov
- The Mayo Clinic website http://www.mayoclinic.org

It is important that you get your online information from reputable and reliable sources. There are many websites that supply false information, give patients unrealistic expectations, and make suggestions that do more harm than good. Learning all you can about your disease empowers you to take charge of your illness instead of being controlled by it.

Your Turn

1. What do you need to change about your mindset as preparation for considering ways to improve your fibromyalgia symptoms? Write down three things you need to focus on while you implement practical priorities to improve your health.
2. If it has been more than a year since you have had any type of laboratory evaluation, make an appointment with your physician to have a checkup and discuss what laboratory work needs to be done. Ask specifically about tests to rule out vitamin deficiencies and thyroid disease. Ask your doctor for recommendations for other tests that might reveal secondary causes for some of your fibromyalgia symptoms. Write out your plan for getting laboratory evaluation, date lab work is done, and the test results.
3. What is your personal spiritual touchstone? Where do you go and what do you do to feel closer to God or to get in touch with your spiritual side? Has your faith been impacted by your illness? How? What can you do to get back to the place that feeds your soul?

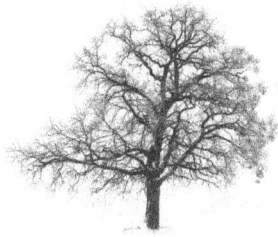

Priority 3: Deal with Depression

DURING THE FIRST year after I was diagnosed with fibromyalgia, I woke up every morning hoping I would finally feel better. Instead, I woke up every morning feeling worse than I had the day before. My pain symptoms multiplied and chronic fatigue left me unable to complete routine tasks. I had no idea how to function within the confines of my new normal.

I kept trying anyway. The first October that rolled around after I got sick, Vic and I debated whether or not to attempt our annual fall camping trip. We love to explore the great outdoors in our motorhome during autumn. We decided that maybe a change of scenery would be good for me. I was weary of the view from my recliner in our den.

We made reservations at a campground nestled in the lovely mountains of western North Carolina, packed, and hit the open road. I envisioned tromping through colorful leaves on woodland trails, exploring quaint little towns perched on hillsides, and visiting the workshops of local artisans. Instead, I spent the entire week we were there either piled up on the couch inside our motorhome or sitting in a chair outside wrapped up in a blanket staring at the mountains off in the distance.

Toward the end of the week, I made an attempt to leave the campground. I love waterfalls. There was one nearby I wanted to see that was located a short 300 yards from the trailhead. I thought that I would be able to accomplish such a tiny walk. I put on my hiking boots, filled my water bottle, and we drove to the trailhead parking lot. I got out of the car and managed to walk about ten yards before I had to sit down on a large boulder. I sat there resting for 15 minutes hoping I would be able to continue. But I couldn't do it. Vic had to help me back to the car. I never did see that waterfall. (Hope note. Three years later, I chased my grandchildren down that same trail and watched that clear mountain stream cascading over the rocky cliffs in those woods.)

I was extremely discouraged by my inability to do things I had always enjoyed. It wasn't long before I tumbled headlong into depression. Depression is a common ancillary symptom with fibromyalgia and other types of chronic illness. My particular depressive pattern stemmed from several factors.

- I was in horrible relentless pain every second of every day. I had been told by multiple doctors that the pain would never go away and that it might get worse. That wasn't exactly conducive to creating hope.
- I had chronic debilitating fatigue that made it difficult for me to complete the most basic tasks of ordinary life. Simply taking a shower often used up my energy allotment for the entire day.
- My usual irritatingly cheerful optimism spiraled into constant pessimism. I lost my sense of self. I didn't know who I was anymore.

I needed to find out more about depression and chronic illness and deal with it before I could focus on finding ways to improve my other symptoms. So, I consulted my internal medicine physician. And, I talked to Vic. In the process, I gathered some helpful facts about depression and how it relates to chronic illness.[3]

Common symptoms that show up with depression are:
- sleep disorders such as insomnia or sleeping all the time
- lack of energy
- constantly feeling blue or in a sad mood
- irritability
- problems focusing
- decreased interest in the normal activities of life
- change in appetite, including eating either more or less than usual
- obsessive thinking in which you focus on one thing that you can't seem to get out of your head

I could check off almost all of these symptoms. I had insomnia, lack of energy, felt constantly sad, had difficulty focusing, and lost interest in the normal activities of life because I was no longer physically able to do any of them. I played the same scene in a constant loop in my mind. Every single day all I could think about was that I was terribly sick with no hope of getting better. This obsessive thinking increased my depressive mood.

If you experience depression as a part of your fibromyalgia symptom pattern, there are several steps you can take to deal with it. Talk to your physician about your depression. Tell him or her about all your present symptoms. Your doctor may advise treatment for depression which may include taking antidepressant medications. These medicines need to be monitored by your doctor. It is important that you keep follow up appointments with your doctor and give him/her an honest assessment of how you are doing. This type of medication often has to be adjusted, increased, or changed over time to treat your specific symptoms.

Additionally, some patients need counseling sessions with a qualified medical professional who is certified in the treatment of depression. If you are not certain how to choose the right clinician, ask your primary care physician for a recommendation. Qualified medical clinicians include psychologists, psychiatrists, licensed certified social workers, counselors, and mental health professionals. Look for someone who specializes in depression and anxiety disorders. Make sure the medical professional you choose has the proper training to treat depression. Ask how long he/she has been in practice, where he/she trained, and what type of certification he/she has. If you do not feel comfortable with your first choice, make an appointment with a different medical professional to get a second opinion. You need to have confidence in both the medical clinician who treats your depression and the physician who treats your fibromyalgia. Be your own advocate. It's important that you have the right medical team to help you cope with chronic illness.

There are several things you can do to help moderate your depressive symptoms. Different things help different people who are dealing with depression. Besides consulting your doctor, taking medication, and consulting a mental health professional that treats depression, you may also benefit from one or more of the following suggestions.
- Find a support group.
- Practice prayer and/or meditation.
- Eat healthy real food, especially fruits, nuts, and vegetables.
- Exercise.
- Get adequate sleep.
- Focus on what you can do instead of on what you can't do.

If anxiety is a component of your depression pattern, making a plan to deal with it can be helpful. Make a list of things that make you feel anxious. Beside each anxiety-inducing event, write down a specific strategy you might implement to deal with it. Here are a few examples

If your anxiety level has increased because you are unable to complete household chores due to your fibromyalgia symptoms, hire someone to clean your house. If this is not financially feasible, enlist the help of friends and family members.

If you are anxious because you can't complete your tasks at work in the same way you could before you got sick, consider what you could conceivably change. Can you reduce your hours? Is it possible to work from home part of the week? Can you find a less stressful job in your field?

Implementing some of the above strategies helped my depression and anxiety. I cut back my hours at work, hired someone to clean my house, made lists of how to deal with specific anxieties, consulted my physician, and focused on what I could still do. Later on, I added exercise to my day, reset my sleep pattern, and changed my diet to emphasize consuming real food. We'll look at these strategies in detail in later chapters of the book.

I implemented these changes slowly over the course of almost a year. In the beginning, one of the things that helped me the most was becoming proactive with my disease. My personal research project to look for ways to improve my symptoms made me feel less helpless and more in control of my illness. I saw a small ray of light in the darkness. Hope was a powerful antidote for my despair.

Dr. Norman Drops By

Because anyone with a chronic illness is naturally going to have some bouts of depression just from the stress of coping with the disease, there is some overlap in the clinical picture of depression and fibromyalgia.

Some patients with fibromyalgia have been misdiagnosed as suffering from only depression because the two diseases have some similar symptom patterns. For example, patients with fibromyalgia often have difficulty sleeping. The sleep disturbances in fibromyalgia include difficulty falling asleep, difficulty staying asleep, waking up in the middle of the night, and waking up unrefreshed. These same sleep problems are also common in depression. However, depression is not a physically painful disease. Fibromyalgia patients commonly have severe pain along with chronic fatigue and sleep disturbances.

There is also a link between inflammation and both diseases.[4] Research indicates that inflammation contributes to the disease process in both fibromyalgia and depression.[5] The research regarding inflammation from toxic environmental chemicals as a suspected cause of fibromyalgia began in the 1990s and continues today.[6]

There are many reasons patients develop depression. It can be caused by physiological triggers such as addictive behaviors, bipolar disease, and other illnesses. Patients with chronic illnesses like fibromyalgia frequently develop depression when they internalize the reality that they may never recover.

However, the most common causes of depression fall into one of three categories. I call these the three S roots of depression: serotonin, season, and situation.

Serotonin
Serotonin is a chemical neurotransmitter in the nervous system. If a patient has low levels of serotonin, it can cause poor brain function that may result in depression. There are antidepressant medications that can be prescribed to help raise the serotonin levels. Some patients respond well to these medications. In other patients, medication by itself does not completely eradicate depressive episodes. Counseling, exercise, increasing the ability to sleep well, and other treatment may also be required to get this type of depression under control. If your doctor thinks your depression is related to your serotonin levels, he will discuss appropriate treatment options with you.

Season
Seasonal depression most often occurs during the gloomy, dark days of winter. Light deprivation during the shorter days of

winter can produce depression in susceptible patients. Patients usually improve with increased exposure to light. You can either increase your exposure to natural light by spending time outside or by spending time underneath an artificial light or lamp that utilizes the same wavelength as sunlight.

Situation

Specific situations can also be a factor in patients who suffer with depression. Situational depression can be caused by such things as grief and loss over the death of a loved one, going through a divorce, losing a job, and having to deal with chronic illness on a daily basis. This type of depression often resolves on its own when the situation resolves. If the situation is not going to change over time, consulting your physician and/or seeing a counselor can be helpful.

There is a unique situational link between depression and spirituality that has the potential to cause collateral damage to people of faith. Common to any form of depression, regardless of the cause, are feelings of guilt, abandonment, and a sense of being unloved. These feelings impact patients with chronic illness both inside and outside of the faith community. It is common for patients to feel a loss of connection to the human race, their own personal spirituality, their belief in the goodness of people, and their own self-worth.

Because my practice was located in the heart of the Bible belt, many of my patients were church-going Christians. Often the feelings of depression they experienced were interpreted in a spiritual context which focused on the patient's relationship with God.

It was not unusual for these patients to feel the guilt of real or imagined sins, abandonment by God, unworthy of having a relationship with God, or feeling unloved by God. Because of this dynamic, much of my time with patients with depression was spent in educating them about the nature and causes of depression. I was also able to offer spiritual counseling as needed to help a person of faith get the proper perspective on the problem.

All illnesses, including depression, have physical, mental, and spiritual aspects. However, and I cannot emphasize this strongly enough, depression is not an indication of spiritual failure due to a lack of faith or a lack of prayer. It is a specific diagnosable disease with a wide variety of treatment options.

I spent a lot of time undoing the harm caused by what well-meaning people said to depressed patients. Sometimes, pastors and fellow church members told a patient that his problem was caused by some sin that he needed to root out and confess. This only added guilt to the depression making the situation worse, even causing some patients to contemplate suicide.

Sometimes a patient was told by other Christians that if she just prayed enough, focused on happy thoughts, and got over feeling blue everything would be fine. Other patients were told that everything was in their heads and they just needed to get over it.

I was constantly astounded at the audacity of people who criticized patients suffering from depression. These folks would never dream of telling someone suffering from a brain tumor to just get over it or advise someone recovering from a stroke to just think happy thoughts and they would be able to walk and speak again.

Depression is an illness just like cancer and heart disease. A qualified healthcare professional is needed to address and treat this illness. Depression is a common component of fibromyalgia and other chronic diseases. It is a normal and valid situation for people of faith who are struggling with a chronic illness to question God and to have doubts about their beliefs. A positive relationship of trust in God can be very therapeutic for a patient suffering from a debilitating disease. But getting back to a place of trust and faith can be a process that takes time for some patients. These patients do not need criticism and advice from people who have no training in how to treat depression. They need support, understanding, and encouragement from their doctors and from the people in their faith community.

Your Turn

1. If you suffer from depression as part of your chronic illness pattern or as a separate issue, consult your physician and plan appropriate treatment. Write down your plan to deal with depression.
2. Taking charge of my illness, doing my own research project, and making lifestyle changes to move toward well-being helped me turn my pessimism into a more optimistic outlook long before my symptoms improved. Write down three things that help you feel more positive about your life.
3. Make a list of things that increase your anxiety level. Write down one specific action you will take to decrease each specific anxiety.

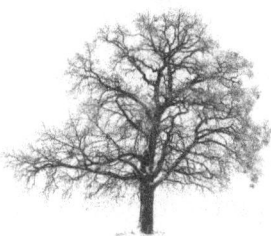

Priority 4: Identify Your Support Network

SINCE CHILDHOOD, I'VE been headstrong, stubborn, opinionated, and independent. That's about what you'd expect from someone who is an Enneagram 8: The Challenger. Before the onslaught of fibromyalgia, I was usually chomping at the bit to take control and confront any problem with a barrage of creative problem-solving tactics until the issue was resolved. Now I stared at all nine Enneagram profiles and didn't see myself in any of them. I needed more number choices. Maybe I was a 0: Completely Defeated, or a 10: Dazed and Confused.

My personal research project indicated that eventually I needed to find ways to create a chemical-free life if I wanted to move toward the possibility of reducing my fibromyalgia symptoms. Thinking about how to deal with this particular problem left me feeling awkward, hesitant, weak, unsure, and full of doubt. I needed to tap into my inner stubborn independent child. But she seemed to be hiding out somewhere far away from my present reality.

It was a good thing that I had a strong support group as I staggered around limping toward change. Vic was my biggest cheerleader and a constant source of information and validation. I was also blessed with a far-flung circle of family and friends who helped me when I was too sick to help myself, encouraged me as I investigated how to get better, and celebrated with me when I found ways to improve my symptoms. It was a gift to know that no matter what happened next, I had a reliable network of family and friends who had my back.

Unfortunately, I also had some exasperating people in my circle of life that hindered me at every turn. Most of these were acquaintances rather than close friends and family.

There are a lot of negative people in this world who have the potential to be just as toxic to our well-being as the harmful chemicals in our environment. Negative people in our circle of life may include coworkers, friends, acquaintances, fellow church members, medical personnel, family members, or opinionated strangers. In order to maximize our potential for creating a healthier life, it is essential to have strategies in place to deal with negative people.

I ran into four specific groups of potentially problematic people.

The Unbelievers

Because fibromyalgia has no obvious outwardly identifiable signs of illness, there were those who refused to believe that I was really sick. They tried to cajole me into going on a shopping trip on days I barely had enough energy to get out of bed. They suggested that I get up and clean my house on days I was having so much pain that it took every ounce of strength I possessed to keep from crying and screaming. They informed me that my fatigue and pain were all in my head and suggested that I just needed to shake it off and move on.

There were those who refused to believe that chemical ingredients in household products, scents, cosmetics, and food have any negative effect on our health whatsoever. Even people who suffer from some type of chronic illness themselves have looked at me with disbelief when I enthusiastically share the health benefits of creating a chemical-free life. Some have flat out said they don't think eliminating chemicals would make a bit of difference and they have refused to change a single thing.

The Know-It-Alls

Some folks are incapable of hearing about any illness without announcing that they have the perfect way to cure the problem. If I would only try this medicine, take this supplement, do what their cousin's husband's next-door neighbor did, I would feel better. I always appreciate hearing other people's stories, learning what helps folks with fibromyalgia feel better, gathering new ideas for healthy living, and discovering ways to boost my immune system. I am thankful for people willing to share their personal experiences about practical ways to cope with the reality of living with a chronic illness.

It is a wonderful thing to share our journeys with one another. This can be a great source of encouragement. However, people who are not sick, have no background knowledge of a particular disease, have not implemented any healthy lifestyle changes themselves, and yet insist they have the perfect solution for my situation are quite exhausting. I hope that the practical strategies shared in this book give you the resources you need to create a chemical-free life, design your own personal healthy living plan, and move toward fibromyalgia recovery. However, I certainly do not have all the answers for every single person and every single chronic illness.

The Polluters

Some people refused to cooperate in my quest to remove chemicals from my environment and diet. They demanded I eat processed food after I learned how harmful it was to my health. They insisted that one bite couldn't hurt me. They were miffed when I declined to taste something they had concocted by dumping things from boxes and cans into a mixing bowl. They arrived at my house drenched in perfume after I politely explained I needed to stay away from scented products. They constantly polluted my environment with the very chemicals I was working hard to eliminate.

The Blockers
There were those folks who threw obstacles into my path. They made negative comments about me and my illness. They found something wrong with every single thing I tried to do to move toward recovery. They discouraged me by their words and actions and attitudes. If I made two-steps forward, it seemed like they felt their mission in life was to push me three steps back.

If you decide to create a chemical-free life to move toward healing, what can you do about those people who are not helping you at all but are, in fact, driving you crazier with each passing day? This depends on who the person is and what the situation is. It is important to remember that you are the one who decides how much control you allow negative people to have in your life. Here are a few ideas.

If your doctor is skeptical that you are really sick, has no experience in treating fibromyalgia or other autoimmune diseases, or has no helpful suggestions regarding your treatment, it is time to look for another doctor.

If your aunt adamantly refuses to quit drenching herself in perfume every time you see her, limit your visits to her home.

If your neighbor constantly puts you down, offers offensive opinions about your condition, or is always negative about your illness, curtail the amount of time you spend with her.

If a stranger makes an inappropriate comment, decide in advance that you are going to smile and be kind even if they are rude. No one has the power to make you feel bad about yourself unless you allow them to do so.

When my disease was at its worst, I always used the handicapped stall in public restrooms because my pain was so severe, I needed to hold on to the grab bars to use the facilities. I was greeted with disapproving stares on more than one occasion when I emerged from the stall because I didn't have a cane or a wheelchair. I always gave those scowling faces the most radiant smile I could muster.

If the discouraging, uncooperative, negative person is a close family member or a coworker and limiting contact is not an option, you may have to try a different approach. Information and patience are two good strategies. The more the problematic person understands about your illness and the things you are trying to do to get better, the more cooperation you may get. This often will not happen overnight so you have to be patient while waiting for that person to see the light.

Ultimately, I had to assume responsibility for my illness, my response to it, and my efforts to move toward recovery. After all, making drastic changes in my lifestyle was my decision, not someone else's. Sometimes I had to miss a party, avoid eating at a certain restaurant, or not attend a family gathering. I recognized that every single person in my life was not required to make changes just because I was making changes.

I hope you have more positive people in your life than negative people. I encourage you to find creative, helpful ways to deal with toxic people as you move toward creating a chemical-free life to improve your symptoms.

Fibromyalgia and other chronic autoimmune diseases have no outwardly obvious symptoms easily identified by others. Your friends, family, and coworkers are not mind readers. They will not know how traumatic it is for you to feel so ill all the time unless you make them aware of what is going on in your life. This is understandable.

What I have difficulty understanding is the number of people I know with this horrible disease who cannot find a competent physician who believes they are sick. I am shocked and astounded at the things I hear from fellow sufferers. They have been told by doctors:

"You are just tired and overworked."

"It is a mental problem. You are not physically sick."

"You are just depressed and feeling blue."

"I can't find a single thing wrong with you."

"I don't believe fibromyalgia exists."

Fortunately, there are also a lot of understanding, caring physicians who listen to their patients, acknowledge their symptoms, and treat them with care and respect. If you have been unlucky enough to have encountered an inadequate doctor, please don't despair and give up. Keep looking. Ask for recommendations from friends and family. Ask other people who have fibromyalgia and chronic autoimmune diseases for physician recommendations. Keep making appointments until you find the right doctor for you.

I have been blessed to have great doctors. I am married to a family physician who is the smartest, kindest, wisest, most caring doctor and human being that I know. (It is possible I am a little biased about this, but I don't think so.) My specialists listened and responded to my questions and concerns. My doctors supported me, encouraged me, and helped me navigate the multilayered realities of dealing with a chronic illness.

Later on, I'm going to explain how I created an environment conducive to promoting health and encourage you to do the same. This will more than likely require you to make a multitude of changes in your lifestyle. So, buckle up and hold on to your hat. And for heaven's sake, find your support group and hold on to these folks with all your might. These are the very people you can count on to keep holding on to you.

Dr. Norman Drops By

It is important for people to have a supportive group of friends and family they can count on in all circumstances. Those who help us when we are sick and encourage us as we create a healthier life exemplify the saying from an old Swedish proverb: "Shared joy is a double joy; shared sorrow is half a sorrow." Do you have people in your life who double your joy and halve your sorrow? Who are the loving, caring, and accepting people in your personal support system? Let's look at four categories of folks that have the potential to support us as we deal with health issues and lifestyle changes.

Family and Friends
The basic support group for most people is family and close friends. These are the people who you naturally most often turn to for understanding and unconditional love. Perhaps you do not have a good relationship with your family, so your close friends become your most ardent supporters. Perhaps you don't have many close friends so your family becomes your primary point of advocacy. You are twice blessed if you have both family and friends who support you and encourage you through all the ups and downs of life.

Healthcare Providers
You should also be able to count on getting support from your physician and his medical staff when you are ill. The primary purpose and goal of your physician and his or her staff is to provide help and healing for the patients in his or her care. Your doctor and staff should create a supportive and caring environment in the office setting. When I was in private practice, the nurses, receptionist, and business office personnel worked together with me to express their care for patients through acts of kindness and concern.

If your physician is one of the negative people in your life, then you need to find another doctor. When I was on the admissions committee for our state medical school, our interviews with prospective medical school students focused on finding applicants whose lives expressed caring and concern for others. This is what you need in a physician. Even if a doctor does not understand fibromyalgia or another chronic illness you are dealing with, at the very least, your doctor should still be a caring, compassionate human being. He or she should either become educated about your disease or refer you to another doctor who is trained in dealing with your specific illness. If you have difficulty finding a supportive physician, I recommend that you look for a qualified therapist, certified social worker, or understanding counselor who will listen to your concerns and help you negotiate the difficult terrain of coping with chronic illness.

Church Congregations
If you are a person of faith, your church may also be a great source of support and comfort for you. Churches, Bible study groups, and prayer groups often are places where people are able to share their lives in a loving setting. This may be a place that you can ask for and receive support from the group in the form of prayer and fellowship. If you feel that you cannot count on your congregation and if the people in your church exude more negative than positive energy, then you may need to consider looking for a more loving, caring faith community.

Advocacy Groups
Some people feel they don't have a single person in their life who they can trust to love them unconditionally and support them as they deal with chronic illness. In this case, you need to look for a support group in your area that can take up the slack from uncaring family and friends. Advocacy groups that have been formed for a specific illness, such as fibromyalgia, cancer,

or heart disease, can also be a great source of support for anyone dealing with a chronic disease. These groups often prove to be great resources for providing education and information regarding your specific illness. Your city may have a fibromyalgia, chronic fatigue, or chronic illness support group you can join. There are fibromyalgia support groups and information forums on Facebook and Twitter. You may want to start a chronic illness support group at your church or community center. Sharing what you are going through with someone who understands is a great encouragement. As you implement lifestyle changes that move you toward the possibility of recovery, sharing methods you discover that help you feel better is a gift that you can pass on to fellow sufferers.

Unfortunately, there are groups of people who will not be supportive of you while you are trying to create a healthier life. If the particular circumstances of your life involve interactions with negative people on a routine basis, there are some specific techniques you can employ in dealing with them.

Avoidance
You may be able to make a choice to simply spend as little time as possible with some negative people. There may be some activities you can eliminate from your life if they include people who make you feel worse about yourself and your illness. You may need to walk away from a club, community group, Bible study class, or other optional activity if there is too much negative energy associated with continued participation. You have the freedom to choose.

In other instances, this will not be possible. If the negative person is a coworker you have to interact with each workday or a close family member you frequently see, avoidance may not be an option. There are many skills you can use to communicate with negative people in a positive way. Two simple methods are to use active listening and "I" statements.

Active Listening

One effective way to deal with negative people is to use a communication technique called active listening. With this technique, you first listen to what the person says. Then instead of arguing with the person or making contradictory obser- vations, you restate what they have just said using different words. If someone says, "I don't see why you can't pull your share of the work load around here. You don't look that sick to me," try this. Instead of getting angry or defensive, respond with, "It sounds like you are upset because I can't do as much work as I could before I was ill. I think I hear you saying that you wonder what the symptoms of my illness are since they are not something you can see." Sometimes, restating what the negative person has said lets them hear how their words sound to you. In any case, it keeps you from being goaded into an argumentative response.

"I" Statements

Another technique is to use "I" statements instead of "you" state- ments. A negative person may say, "I don't think fibromyalgia is a real disease. You are a mental case. It's all in your head." Instead of responding with, "You make me so mad when you say things like that. You don't understand anything. You are just mean and ignorant." try saying, "I feel hurt when someone says fibromyalgia is all in my head. It makes me feel so sad that you don't understand how sick I am. I will be glad to explain my symptoms to you if you would like for me to do that."

Hopefully, using these techniques will help real communi- cation take place and lead to better understanding between you and the difficult people in your life. Having a physician that you trust, the support of your family and friends, and an advocacy group are invaluable resources as you move toward creating a healthier life.

Your Turn

1. Make a list of the people who you think will be the most supportive as you create a healthy living plan to help improve your fibromyalgia symptoms. List specific ways you think these particular people will be supportive.

2. Identify the Unbelievers, Know-It-All, Polluters, and Blockers that you think will be most likely to hinder your attempts to make lifestyle changes. List ways you feel they may hamper your progress in meeting your goal to improve your symptoms.

3. Choose one of the techniques discussed in this chapter that you will use to minimize the hindrances each of the negative people on your list could have on your health goals. Name the person and the technique you plan to use.

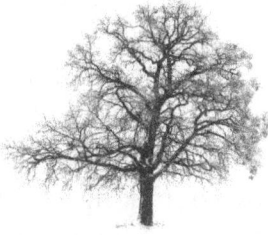

Priority 5: Recognize We Live in a Toxic World

AFTER THE FIRST few months of my personal research project, I had a better understanding of fibromyalgia. I redirected my focus from the problems of my illness to the possibilities for improvement. I faced the fact that chronic illness can cause depression and found ways to deal with it. I had a great support group. I had read several articles along the way about the relationship between exposure to toxic chemicals and chronic illness. I was ready to investigate what I could do to detoxify my life.

I was shocked when I discovered how many potentially harmful chemical ingredients are used to manufacture fragrance, cleaners, household products, processed food, cosmetics, personal grooming items, and other ordinary things that I used every day.[7]

We live in an extremely toxic world. I had a lot of questions. Where are the most toxic substances found? Why did I not know about this before? What could I do about any of it?

Where are the most toxic substances found?

I was vaguely aware there were toxic substances floating around in the atmosphere. I read the news a few years back about the lead in the water in Flint, Michigan. I saw smog choking the air in every large metropolitan area I visited. I heard people on talk shows blathering about coal dust, industrial pollution, and pesticides.

I may have glanced at an article or two in the waiting room of some medical office or the other about harmful ingredients used to create cosmetics and cleaning products. I heard somebody on some television program going on and on about the dangers of eating too much processed food. But I shrugged, rolled my eyes, and wandered off to look for the bag of chocolate chip cookies.

As it turns out, I should have been paying more attention. Thousands of unhealthy chemicals and additives are used in the mass production of food. Grocery store shelves are filled with boxes and cans and bottles of items that would never have been considered safe for human consumption before the industrialization of food. I ate tons of this stuff mindlessly for decades because it never occurred to me that items available for purchase in my neighborhood grocery store might be harmful to my health.[8]

And it's not just processed food. Tons of potentially harmful ingredients are used to manufacture cosmetics, personal grooming items, and household cleaners. I was bombarded by hundreds of toxic chemicals every single day. I was clueless to this reality for decades.

Why didn't I know about this before?

In the course of my personal research project, I asked myself about a thousand times how in the world I had remained so oblivious about the impact of toxic chemical exposure. There are probably a hundred reasons but, for me, it boiled down to three main factors.

- Habit
  I was over fifty when my fibromyalgia diagnosis motivated me to consider the possible dangers of chemical exposure. And I wouldn't have started looking, even then, if this chronic illness hadn't upended my ability to function normally. I was accustomed to using the same cleaning products and personal care items I had used for decades. I liked eating things that came in boxes and bags. Familiarity is comfortable and change is hard.
- Naïve Trust
  I had some vague subconscious idea that if an item was available for sale in my local supermarket or big box store, it must be okay to use or consume. They (whoever they are) would certainly not be allowed to market and sell something that might harm me.
- Selective Blindness
  When it came right down to it, I wasn't the slightest bit interested in finding out the truth. That might require action, disruption in my routine, and (gasp) significant change in the way I did life. It was easier to ignore the truth than to deal with it.

What could I do about it?

I'm not an expert. I am just an ordinary woman who looked for realistic ways to improve my health. Over time a plan emerged and took shape. I identified specific harmful substances, developed strategizes to detoxify my body and my home, and made lifestyle changes that truly changed my life.

The processed food industry, cosmetic companies, fragrance developers, and household products manufacturers may spew toxic ingredients into my everyday world with little regard for how this compromises my health; but I don't have to use products that are full of toxic ingredients. I get to decide how I spend my money. There were many safer options made with nontoxic ingredients for every single chemically laden thing I needed to replace. Nobody was twisting my arm making me drink diet soda, eat boxes of cookies, spritz toxic chemical cleaners all over my house, and slather preservative filled lotions and makeup onto my skin.

I have control over what goes into and onto my body. Some multinational corporation that measures me as a profit percentage doesn't get to decide what I buy. Once I internalized the truth that I held the power to choose, everything changed.

Dr. Norman Drops By

When Kathy and I began to explore possible causes and treatment options for her illness, it soon became apparent that there was a correlation between the disease process and harmful substances in the environment. Exposure to environmental toxins has been linked to illnesses including fibromyalgia, asthma, chronic sinus infections, heart disease, diabetes, almost every autoimmune disease, and many types of cancer.[9] Avoiding exposure to harmful chemicals in things you use every day including highly processed foods, cosmetics, personal care products, and household cleaners is essential if you want to create a healthier life for yourself and your family.

It is helpful to understand the link between chemical exposure and autoimmune diseases. It is quite probable that the multisystemic symptoms of fibromyalgia are linked to some type of chronic chemical exposure which acts as a poison affecting the entire body.[10]

There are thousands of chemicals in our environment which are manmade. People were not exposed to these chemicals in the past because these chemicals did not exist. Scientists and researchers continue to debate the level of toxicity of chemicals and additives used to manufacture processed food and household products. Kathy didn't wait for the debate to be resolved. She eliminated every product made with ingredients that might negatively impact her well-being. This small sample will give you an idea of the kinds of harmful substances we are exposed to on a daily basis and the potential they have for compromising our health.

- Artificial Food Coloring has been linked to the onset of various types of cancer including thyroid, adrenal, bladder, kidney, and brain cancers.[11]
- High Fructose Corn Syrup (HFCS) is added to hundreds of processed foods including bread, canned vegetables, candy, cereal, condiments, and cookies. HFCS may contain contaminants like mercury depending on the source of the HFCS. This additive is not regulated by the Federal Drug Administration (FDA) or any other oversight committee. The food products that are the least nutritious are the ones most likely to contain HFCS. It raises triglyceride levels and causes overeating, which leads to increased weight and a wide variety of health problems. [12]
- Nitrates and Nitrites are food preservatives used in bacon, lunch meat, and hot dogs. They are suspected to be a possible causal agent in colon cancer and in metabolic syndrome which can lead to the onset of diabetes.[13]
- Formaldehyde is used in the manufacture of some types of glue, cleaners, cosmetics, and even in some brands of baby wipes. It can cause headaches, rashes on the skin, breathing difficulties, fatigue, and stomach upset. It has been linked to some types of cancer.[14]
- Bisphenol A (BPA) and Phthalates are used to make lots of commonly used products including plastic containers, shower curtains, and backpacks. They are used as stabilizers in the manufacture of products that contain fragrance including perfumes, soaps, and lotions. These chemicals can disrupt the normal function of the

endocrine, immune, and reproductive systems. They are linked as causal agents to asthma, chronic illness, and some types of cancer.[15]

- Butylated hydroxyanisole (BHA) and butylated hydroxytoluene (BHT) are used as preservatives in processed foods, moisturizers, and lipstick. They have been linked to a variety of health problems ranging from skin rashes to some types of cancer.[16]
- Pesticides are designed for the sole purpose of killing living things. It is logical that the ingredients used to make them are toxic. Exposure to pesticides has been linked to a variety of cancers, certain types of birth defects, and disruption of the nervous and endocrine systems.[17]

The body is designed to stay healthy. It constantly fights this chemical intrusion with its immune system trying to rid itself of these foreign invaders. This causes inflammation which is one possible cause for the onset of a fibromyalgia pattern. Widespread chemical exposure is also a probable cause for the onset of many other disease processes. This exposure diminishes the effective functioning of the immune system and compromises overall health. You need to minimize exposure to toxic chemicals to cope with chronic illness, boost the immune system, prevent diseases, and create the healthiest life possible.

Your Turn

1. On a scale of one to ten, what is your current awareness level of the amount of potentially harmful chemicals you are exposed to each day? Write a brief note about how habit, naïve trust, and/or selective blindness impact your reaction to the reality that chemicals are harmful to your health.

2. Grab three processed food products from your pantry. Choose one can, one box, one sweet treat. Read the ingredients labels. Are any of them made with artificial food coloring, BHA, HFCS, nitrates/nitrites, and/or some other chemical you don't recognize? List each product and the potentially toxic substances you found on the ingredients label.

3. Look at the label on your favorite cosmetic or personal grooming product. What ingredients are in it? Does it contain fragrance, phthalates, BPA, BHT, BHA, formaldehyde, or other ingredients you don't recognize? Write down the product and list any potentially harmful substances you found on the ingredients label.

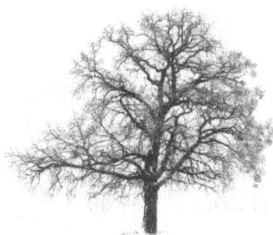

Priority 6: Remove Scented Products from Your Home

DECIDED TO LOOK for ways to create a chemical-free life to see if it would help improve my fibromyalgia symptoms. I didn't have a clue about the best strategies for designing a practical plan, but I kept scrolling through cyberspace anyway. I found random new facts each day. During the first few months of my personal research project, there was no change in my two most prominent physical symptoms: excruciating pain and debilitating fatigue. However, there was a noticeable shift in my mental and emotional state.

I felt more positive than I had in over a year. Taking control of my own medical education by gathering information made me feel less helpless. I was only reading and I had no idea what I was looking for, but I hoped I would recognize the path I needed to follow when I finally found it. It was extremely encouraging to actively look for possibilities rather than just give up and give in to my pain and fatigue. Hope was a powerful thing after months of crushing despair.

After I read the article about the danger of volatile organic compounds (VOCs) in scented products, I thought it might be possible that exposure to toxic substances in fragrance and other household products I used every day was a factor in my fibromyalgia symptom pattern. Environmental chemicals are harmful to everyone. It made sense that exposure to toxic chemicals would be particularly toxic for folks with any type of chronic illness.

I read so much about the thousands of harmful chemicals we are exposed to from multiple sources that I felt like I was in a constant state of imminent danger. I knew I needed to do something to escape the toxicity; but I wasn't sure how to accomplish this.

I had stumbled across one tiny speck of specific useful information: the chemicals in fragrance are harmful to our health.[18] I stopped reading and decided to see what happened if I eliminated scented products from my home. This seemed like a logical place to start since there is absolutely no need to use anything that contains fragrance or scent.

From the very beginning of my quest to improve my health, I had two primary criteria.

- I would try only those things that could cause no harm. I certainly didn't want to do anything that would make my situation worse.
- Everything I tried had to be practical. I didn't have the energy or inclination to try a bunch of complicated hoopla.

Eliminating all scented products from my home environment was not dangerous so I had the do no harm thing covered. It seemed like a practical place to start. As I switched gears from just reading to actually taking action, I was initially overwhelmed by the daunting task of making changes in my lifestyle. I felt horrible from my illness. I didn't know if I had even a smidgen of surplus energy to implement change. Nevertheless, I took a deep breath and summoned the resolve to take one small step at a time.

The strategies I share in this book didn't fall into my lap in completed form. I didn't even know what the completed form would eventually look like. I discovered things randomly and bit by bit. Sometimes I spent weeks accomplishing one small change. Sometimes, I didn't make any changes at all for a month. It was a clumsy one step forward and three steps back kind of dance as I lurched toward creating a healthier reality. And the first part of the dance concerned scented products.

Products that contain scent are dangerous, not because of the fragrance produced, but because most scented products use volatile organic compounds (VOCs) to bind the scent to the products. The words volatile organic compounds and/or the initials VOC may not be listed on the product label. However, if you see the word fragrance or scent in the ingredients list, that means that VOCs were used in the manufacturing process to bind the scent to the product. In addition, products that contain fragrance often contain other toxic artificially manufactured ingredients, as well. The chemicals used to produce fragrance, even when we are exposed to small amounts of them, can cause a wide variety of reactions including itchy eyes, irritated skin, headaches, dizziness, and constant fatigue.[19]

Some scented products are easy to identify: perfume, cologne, scented candles, and air fresheners. I also found some not so obvious products that contain fragrance: cosmetics, personal care items, toilet tissue, cleaners, and laundry detergent. I morphed into a woman on a mission. I ransacked cabinets and cupboards and discarded every cleaning product, personal grooming item, cosmetic, container, box, and bottle that had the word fragrance or scent listed as an ingredient.

Artificial air fresheners, plug-in scents, synthetically scented candles, and perfume are particularly dangerous because they are airborne. They are full of harmful chemicals that you inhale every time you use them. Anything you breathe in through your lungs eventually ends up in your bloodstream where it circulates to every organ in your body with the potential to cause damage on a cellular level in every part of your body.

This not only impacts you personally, it also affects everyone who lives in your home. Our children, grandchildren, visiting friends, and even our pets, are exposed to the toxic ingredients in everything we use on a routine basis in our homes.

Eliminating scented products from my home environment was just the beginning. I'm glad I didn't know that then or I might have been paralyzed into inactivity. I was exposed to many other types of toxic chemicals on a daily basis in cleaning products, personal care items, and other household products I had used for years. I would eventually change almost everything in my everyday ordinary life. For now, getting scented products out of my home was enough.

Dr. Norman Drops By

Products that contain scent are only one category of potentially toxic household products. There are many types of toxic chemicals. There are unsafe chemicals in the environment and in processed foods that contribute to a wide range of symptoms in a wide range of illnesses. To maintain a healthy lifestyle, these chemicals need to be eliminated from your home environment. Two things to consider: VOCs are dangerous and you have the power to control your own health.

VOCs Are Dangerous
Volatile organic compounds (VOCs) are one of the most prevalent categories of unsafe chemicals. Products that include fragrance as an ingredient usually also contain VOCs. Household products and personal care items that contain the VOCs found in fragrance need to be eliminated from the home environment to optimize health.

There is a big difference between common nonvolatile organic compounds, which generally are safe, and volatile organic compounds (VOCs), which are not. Organic compounds are combinations of elements that contain carbon atoms. For example, vinegar is an organic compound consisting of the elements carbon, hydrogen, and oxygen. Vinegar is obviously not a dangerous compound.

Volatile organic compounds can cause reactions in your body that make your health deteriorate. Volatile compounds, such as acetone and formaldehyde, rapidly become vapors at room temperature. Any product that includes fragrance as an ingredient is problematical because scents are dissolved in VOCs so that as the VOCs evaporate, they carry the scent with them. The VOCs are then easily inhaled through the lungs and immediately enter the bloodstream where they are carried to every organ in the body and have the potential to damage every organ in the body.

VOCs are widely used as ingredients in household products such as paints, cleaning supplies, perfume, scented products, permanent markers, wax, aerosol propellants, and craft materials including glues and adhesives. Anytime you use products that contain VOCs, you put your health and the health of your children at risk because the vapors they produce are so easily inhaled into the body.

Some VOCs, such as benzene which is known to cause cancer, and methylene chloride which causes carbon monoxide poisoning, have been banned from use by manufacturers due to their fatal toxicity. Unfortunately, the effects of most VOCs have not been studied sufficiently to know all of their side effects, especially the long-term effects. What is known is that VOCs are a factor in the etiology of asthma, headaches, allergic skin reactions, shortness of breath, nausea and vomiting, fatigue, and dizziness. With exposure to VOCs there is also an increased risk of developing cancer and a risk of damage to the liver, kidneys, brain, and the nervous system.[20]

You Can Take Charge of Your Own Health Outcome

Removing these toxic chemicals from your environment is essential to maintaining your health, preventing illnesses, and giving your body the optimum chance to recover if you are already ill. When I was in private practice, I recommended that patients avoid scented products, especially if they or their family members suffered from recurrent respiratory conditions such as sinus infections, asthma, or allergic rhinitis. The patients who followed this advice, in conjunction with other treatment recommendations, had decreased episodes of these types of disease. Other patients with a similar symptom pattern refused to stop using perfume, air freshener, scented plug-ins, and the like. Their treatment outcomes were worse and they continued to have a high rate of recurrence of respiratory illnesses, sinus infection, and the like.

It is an interesting clinical dynamic that some patients have the mindset that when they are sick all they need to do is go to the doctor and get a shot or prescription. They feel that illnesses occur randomly and have nothing to do with their lifestyles and choices. In some instances, this is a fair assessment. The disease occurs from exposure to a germ or other pathogen and medication is needed for healing.

However, some conditions are linked to lifestyle choices. In these cases, there are things individuals can do to promote healing and prevent illnesses. One simple strategy is to avoid using all products that contain scent or fragrance as an ingredient. Scented products laden with VOCs have a known impact as a causal agent in the etiology of many respiratory conditions and other disease patterns.

There are numerous chemicals to which we are exposed every day that have unknown effects on our bodies. In fact, each year there are literally hundreds of new chemicals added to our food, household products, and to the environment that have not been tested by any regulatory agency such as the Food and Drug Administration (FDA) or the Environmental Protection Agency (EPA). Chemicals are allowed to be added to products with no knowledge as to their possible detrimental effects. So, you have to be your own regulatory agency and police your own environment. Eliminating products made with hazardous chemicals from your home is a smart strategy for creating a healthier life. Eliminating all scented products is a good place to start.

Your Turn

1. The top three most commonly used products with fragrance in most homes are air fresheners, scented candles, and perfume. If you have any of these in your home, throw them away. List the items you tossed, the room where you found each one, and the date you removed each item from your home.

2. Go grab your favorite cosmetic product or personal care item. Read the ingredients label on this one product. If fragrance is listed as an ingredient, the next time you go shopping, look for a scent-free replacement. Write down the item, the date you threw it out, and the scent-free product you bought as a replacement. Check your other cosmetics as you have time. A simple way to do this is to check the ingredients label as you use up each product. If your current brand contains fragrance, buy a scent-free version when it is time to purchase the product again.

3. Pick two cleaning items you currently use. Check the labels to see if fragrance is an ingredient. The next time you go shopping, look for a scent-free substitute. Check your other cleaning products as you have time. A simple way to do this is to check the ingredients label as

you use up each product. If your current brand contains fragrance, buy a scent-free version when it is time to purchase the product again. Write down the item, the date you threw it out, and the scent-free product you bought as a replacement.

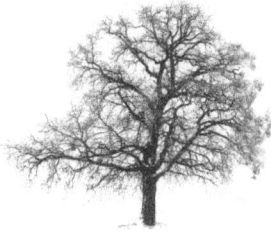

Priority 7: Exchange Harmful Household Products for Safer Ones

AFTER I ELIMINATED all products that contained fragrance from my home, I noticed some small encouraging improvements in the way I felt. Fibromyalgia can cause dozens of odd symptoms. In addition to my two primary symptoms of widespread muscle and joint pain and debilitating chronic fatigue; over the course of my illness, I experienced other symptoms including numbness and tingling in my extremities, dizziness, balance issues, insomnia, and shortness of breath. Although my pain level was still severe and the chronic fatigue was awful, my dizziness and balance were better and the breathing issues had completely resolved.

I was thrilled that eliminating scented products from my home seemed to correlate with some welcomed improvement in my symptom pattern. It motivated me to continue my research. I looked for other possible sources of toxic chemical exposure and specific lifestyle changes that might help me feel better. It would have been awesome if eliminating scented products from my home had completely eliminated every one of my symptoms.

Fibromyalgia syndrome is a complicated illness composed of a broad spectrum of complex symptoms. It made sense that finding ways to improve might require making more than one small lifestyle change.

Different people react in different ways to the idea of change. I've noticed an interesting dynamic in discussion threads on online fibromyalgia forums. Someone suggests a specific food to eat, food to avoid, lifestyle change to make, chemical to eliminate, exercise regimen, or another lifestyle change that has proved helpful to that person. A reader tries one, just one, of these ideas, has no immediate results, gives up after a few days, disparages the person and the suggestion, and then retreats into hopelessness.

We are unique and intricate human beings. There are unique and intricate causes for fibromyalgia syndrome and unique and intricate symptom patterns. My road to recovery was unique and intricate. Yours will be too. It took a combination of lifestyle changes before I noticed significant improvement. Patience, persistence, and perseverance were necessary as I continued my research.

Since removing products made with VOC laden fragrance from my home improved a few of my symptoms, during the next phase of my personal research project, I looked for other sources of exposure to harmful chemicals known to adversely affect our health.

I was overwhelmed by the sheer volume of toxic chemicals we are exposed to from multiple sources on a daily basis. There are thousands of chemicals in the water, in the air, in stores, in houses, and in office buildings. Unless I could magically transform myself into a toxic-substance- eradicating- superhero, there was not much I could do about the harmful chemicals in the general environment. I focused my energy on limiting my vulnerability in the place where I had the most control: my own home.

Once upon a time (BF: Before Fibro), I gave little thought to the ingredients that companies use to manufacture common products I use every day for cleaning and personal care.

The truth is there aren't a lot of laws that govern the ingredients companies are allowed to use in the manufacturing process. The laws that do exist are affected by the number of lobbyists angling for a particular industry to circumvent those laws, the platform of the political party currently in office, and the relative power of activists and advocates for chemical-free living in any given year.

It was unrealistic to expect the government, industries, or huge corporations to look out for my health and well-being. That's my job. It was an empowering moment when I realized that I have the leverage every single day to choose a chemical-free life. No one can force me to use toxic products. They can make them. I don't have to buy them.

There are so many chemicals in so many things. I became a zealous label reader. Many of the ingredient names were unrecognizable and unpronounceable. Several chemicals showed up on every list of potentially harmful substances I found: VOCs in the form of added fragrance, formaldehyde, phthalates, preservatives, and petroleum derivatives.

In addition, I discovered there was a significant problem related to dust. Dust?! When I was little, I was entranced by watching dust motes dance in the sunbeams streaming through the windows. Those interesting little motes are very efficient at gathering up every single particle of chemical residue from products I use in my home. As long as the dust stays, each chemical particle clinging to the motes stays.[21]

As I looked for the most practical ways to exchange harmful household products for safer ones, I found that I got the most exposure to harmful chemicals from three categories of things that I used on a daily basis: scented products, cleaning products, and cosmetics/personal care items. I had already dealt with scented products. I was ready to see what I could do about the other two.

Cleaning Products

Cleaning products were a big source of exposure to chemicals in my home. They contain toxic ingredients that I inhaled, touched, got on my skin, and spread onto surfaces all over my house. Some of them may be good at removing dirt and grime but that is counterproductive to creating a healthier home when they leave harmful chemical residue behind every single time they are used.

Most commercially manufactured household products contain harmful ingredients. There are many safer alternatives. I do a lot of laundry so I was thrilled to find there are laundry detergents free of perfume and dyes. One of my favorite laundry discoveries is organic wool dryer balls. I use them in place of fabric softeners and dryer sheets, both of which contain fragrances and chemicals. I toss a couple into the dryer with a load of clothes to reduce wrinkles. They are completely natural and nontoxic. An added bonus is they reduce the time it takes to dry a load of clothes.

There are organic versions of many household cleaners made by a wide variety of companies. Due to an increased interest in healthy chemical-free living, many of the safer versions can be found at ubiquitous big box stores including Walmart, Costco, and Target, and online retailers like Amazon.

Another option for removing harmful chemical cleaning products from my home was making my own cleaners using natural ingredients. My favorite natural ingredient for making my own cleaning products is white vinegar. I buy the least expensive brand at discount stores in huge containers and get a ton of cleaning power for my money. I make my own shower cleaner, toilet bowl cleaner, tile floor cleaner, all-purpose cleaning spray, and more. Check out Appendix I for recipes for household cleaners, pest removers, and other household products that you can make from vinegar, baking soda, and other nontoxic ingredients you probably already have stashed away in your kitchen.

Cosmetics and Personal Care Items

I use makeup and personal care items every day. I was dismayed to learn what is in products I slather on my skin. The Federal Drug Administration (FDA) and the United States Department of Agriculture (USDA) have some input into product labeling but there is no one oversight board to regulate the cosmetic industry. The word natural can be used by any manufacturer on any item. There are a few FDA and USDA regulations for labeling a product as certified 100% organic but that only involves agricultural ingredients. Companies can say a product is made with organic ingredients if it is composed of at least 70% organically certified ingredients, even if the remaining 30% is known to be toxic.[22]

Discovering which toxic ingredients were in the products I currently used and finding an acceptable nontoxic replacement was an ongoing project. I was several months into this process when the gray roots on my then beautiful red hair began to show. I had the phone in my hand to call my stylist for an appointment to refresh my color when it occurred to me that if I wanted to create a chemical-free life, it was probably not a good idea to keep dumping dye on my scalp every month. I had been coloring my hair for so long, I wasn't sure what my natural color was anymore. I let the color grow out and discovered I have chestnut brown har with lots of natural silvery highlights.

I ditched the hair coloring and checked out my other personal grooming supplies and cosmetics. Many types of makeup are a problem, not only because they contain scents that are added using VOCs, but because they may also contain BHA preservatives, coal tar, petroleum derivatives, phthalates, parabens, formaldehyde, mercury, lead, and a lot of other toxic ingredients that have been linked to the onset of autoimmune diseases, disruption of the endocrine system, and some types of cancer.

Because the cosmetics industry regulates itself, consumers need to understand how to choose safer makeup options. One good resource is The Skin Deep Database website http://www.ewg.org/skindeep where you can look up the ingredients in your favorite cosmetics and find a numerical rating for how safe or toxic each one is.

There are brands of hypoallergenic scent free makeup and organic personal care products. If you can't find a completely organic version you like, shampoo and soap that are clear or white tend to contain fewer chemicals than those that have color. You can purchase natural shampoos, soaps, and deodorants that are made without toxic ingredients. Replacing products that come in an aerosol spray with a different version, such as a pump bottle or cream, reduces your exposure to the chemicals used in aerosol propellant.

It can be a daunting task to replace household products, cleaning products, cosmetics, and personal care items you have always used with safer versions. In order to not feel completely overwhelmed, I paced myself by making one small change at a time as I worked toward the goal of getting potentially harmful chemicals out of my home.

I read the labels on everything I routinely used. I found VOCs, fragrance. phthalates, and other harmful chemicals listed as an ingredient in laundry detergent, cleaning products, makeup, bath soap, deodorant, hand lotion, hairspray, and more.

There are several smartphone apps that are helpful tools for learning what is in cleaners, household products, and cosmetics you use each day. Two of my favorites are Detox Me and EWGs Healthy Living. You can find a list of other apps and online resources in Appendix III.

I used the apps and websites and read ingredients labels to learn what was in the products I chose to use. I minimized my risk of exposure to toxic substances in ordinary products I used every day by doing three things.

- I got rid of household products made almost entirely from harmful chemicals. There are hundreds of potentially harmful ingredients in products. I had to start somewhere. I began by eliminating products that contained the five most commonly used toxic ingredients: formaldehyde, BPA, BHA, BHT, and phthalates. I got rid of commercially produced pesticides that are made with toxic chemicals designed to kill.

- I replaced toxic products with safer versions. I make a lot of household cleaning products and pest removers myself. You can find recipes for some of these in Appendix 1. There are a number of companies that make cleaning products and personal care items that are manufactured with fewer toxic ingredients. There are makeup brands that use at least some organic ingredients. You still have to be careful. Companies that market themselves as organic may still use some unsafe chemicals. I was cautious as I looked for safer options. A company can use the word *natural* to describe just about anything. I read labels so that I would know exactly what was in the things I chose to use and I chose to use a safer version of everything.

- I dust and vacuum frequently. This is not a cleaning issue. It is a health issue. Toxic chemicals cling to dust particles. I don't use liquid or spray products full of chemicals when dusting. I use a plain microfiber dusting wand or a microfiber cloth that contains no added cleansers or fragrances. I use a microfiber or cloth dust mop with no added chemicals to keep the dust off of hardwood floors.

I eventually tossed every cleaning item, lipstick, lotion, and other product that listed preservatives, fragrance, formaldehyde, or other toxic substances as an ingredient. I got rid of all pesticides. I purchased or made natural cleaners, hypoallergenic makeup, and natural pest removers.

I would have been overwhelmed to think I had to completely change everything in my life as fast as I could go. I would never have survived such a grueling pace. I had a system. Instead of trying to go through my entire house at once, I checked the ingredients labels on products as I used them. If harmful chemicals were listed on the ingredients label, the next time I went shopping I looked for a less toxic substitute for one or two of the products I needed to replace.

Each time I decided which nontoxic option I liked best and switched to a safer version, I eliminated another toxic chemical from my home. This strategy met my criteria for making changes. It was not harmful and it was something practical that eventually I could accomplish. I decided to create a chemical-free home environment and then I took all the time I needed to figure out exactly how I needed to do it.

I share information and resources with you in this book so that you can create your own personalized chemical-free life and move toward a healthier reality. There are lots of options in this chapter. Choose what works best for you. I like making my own household cleaners. You may prefer buying commercially made versions of products you need that are less toxic than the brands you currently use. I like using organic wool dryer balls. They work great for me here in the humid south. One of my manuscript beta readers had a problem with wool dryer balls causing increased static in the low humidity area where she lives. She found a nontoxic brand of dryer sheets. The goal is not to duplicate my version of a chemical-free life, but to create your own using what works best for you and your lifestyle.

It took several months for me to find everything I needed to change and to settle on an appropriate substitute. It was totally worth the time and effort. Six weeks after I completed the process of exchanging harmful household products for safer ones, my fibromyalgia pain decreased from constant and excruciating to intermittent and bearable.

Looking back, I think it simply took time to detoxify my body. I still had some pain in my muscles and joints, but the pain was far less severe than it had been previously. On a scale of one to ten my pain had stayed at level ten since I had been diagnosed with fibromyalgia. Now it was down to level five most of the time. I still had some days of pain flares when my pain shot back up to the excruciating range; but I now also had some days that were relatively pain free.

Although, the chronic fatigue component of my fibromyalgia pattern had not shown any improvement yet, it was tremendously encouraging to have less pain. I was on the right track. There were more clues out there just waiting to be found. I still had a lot to learn and more changes were on the horizon.

Dr. Norman Drops By

When I was in private practice, patients made appointments at my office for preventive health screenings, treatment of an acute accident or illness, and checkups related to long term chronic illnesses. Often the outcome of these various types of encounters was directly related to a patient's expectations for results. Some correlations were obvious and factual.

Acute illnesses and acute accidents were the area where the patient's expectations most often aligned with mine. If a patient arrived at the office because of an accident, the expectation was that the injuries resulting from the accident would be appropriately treated by me and my staff. If treatment was beyond the scope of my office, the patient would be sent to an appropriate specialist or trauma center. I stitched cuts, debrided wounds, and x-rayed broken bones. I arranged ophthalmology consults for patients with serious eye injuries and sent those with complicated fractures to the nearest orthopedic group.

Similarly, patients who arrived for treatment of an acute illness, such as an upper respiratory infection that was going around that week, expected that I would be aware of this illness in the community and prescribe an appropriate medication and a treatment plan. And this expectation was usually fulfilled. Medicine was given. Rest and recuperation instructions were explained. And the illness resolved as both the patient and I expected it would.

However, for both preventive care and treatment of long-term chronic illnesses the scenario was often quite different. For preventive care, I knew that the patient had the best opportunity for staying healthy if he or she ate healthy food, exercised, didn't smoke, didn't abuse prescription medications, limited alcohol intake, and followed the recommended schedule for laboratory blood work analysis and routine checkups.

Most of my patients were compliant with preventive care plans because they wanted to stay healthy. However, there were always a small number of patients who didn't want to do any of that. They ate whatever they wanted, refused to exercise, continued to smoke, never came in for checkups, and neglected all recommended laboratory analysis. They wanted to have the same outcome as patients who were compliant with preventive care recommendations, but that was an unrealistic expectation. Most of the time my patients and I had the same goals for staying healthy, but sometimes there was a conflicting opinion on the best way to reach these goals.

There was a similar dynamic for patients with chronic illnesses. For example, I knew that a patient with diabetes needed to keep his or her blood sugar under control at a safe level. This often required modifying their diet, taking medications, exercise, and weight loss. All of my patients with diabetes wanted their blood sugar to stay at a safe level but some of them didn't want to change what they ate, lose weight, exercise, or take medication. The outcome for their diabetes management never met my expectations or theirs as long as they refused to change their lifestyle.

Fibromyalgia is a complicated chronic illness. We know more about it now than when I was in practice. Pain receptors in the body and the patient's response to pain are a factor. Patients with fibromyalgia have increased levels of inflammation throughout the body. There is growing evidence that exposure to harmful chemicals is a factor in the ongoing fibromyalgia symptoms of pain, fatigue, dizziness, nausea, gastrointestinal issues, and the other multiple symptoms of the disease.

In addition to playing a role in the fibromyalgia syndrome pattern, exposure to potentially toxic chemicals has been linked to the etiology of a wide array of chronic and long-term illnesses including asthma, cancer, heart disease, immune deficiency diseases, kidney disease, and more.[23]

Chemicals that have the potential to cause toxic reactions include, but are not limited to, formaldehyde, petroleum-based derivatives, artificial dyes, and preservatives. Read the ingredients labels on things you use every day. If you don't recognize an ingredient, the chances are good that your immune system won't recognize it either. The cycle of compromising your health continues with every exposure to every toxic substance.

You can help manage your preventive healthcare and increase the chances for your chronic illness symptoms to improve by avoiding products that are manufactured with toxic chemicals. You can change your outcome if you are willing to change your lifestyle.

Your Turn

1. Read the ingredients label on your laundry detergent, stain remover, and fabric softener. If fragrance, formaldehyde, Bisphenol A (BPA), phthalates, BHA, or BHT is listed as an ingredient, toss that product and find a safer

substitute. Most products in aerosol cans contain toxic substances in the propellants. Replace aerosols with a liquid or pump spray version. List the products you found that contained harmful ingredients, the date you threw each one away, and the safer alternative you purchased as a replacement.

2. Stop using chemical pesticides. Buy chemical-free pest removers. Check out nontoxic ant killer, weed killer, and other pest removers you can make from nontoxic ingredients in Appendix I. List the chemical pesticides you removed from your home, the date you tossed each one out, and the safer replacement you purchased or made.

3. Pick three makeup items you currently use: foundation, powder, blush, eye shadow, mascara, lipstick, etc. Check each one on the Skin Deep Database website at http://www.ewg.org/skindeep or on EWGs Healthy Living smartphone app to find its safety rating. If any of the three makeup items you check have a high toxicity rating, toss it and replace it with a safer version. List the toxic makeup products you found, the harmful chemicals in each one, and the safer replacement you bought.

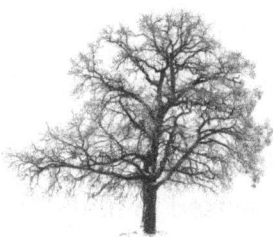

Priority 8: Eliminate Most Processed Food from Your Diet

HAVE A LONG and loving relationship with processed food. I am a huge junk food junkie. I don't have a sweet tooth. I have a whole mouth full of sweet teeth. I love cookies, cake, pie, and candy. So, obviously, when I read that there are harmful chemicals in almost all highly processed foods, including packaged sweets, I had no problem at all with immediately eradicating all processed food from my diet. After all, I'm a responsible, sensible adult and so, I, umm...

Actually, my reaction to this news was more along the lines of: "There are harmful chemicals in packaged cookies and candy? Noooooooooo! I've already turned my normal daily routine upside down, changed every one of my cleaning products, and completely altered my personal care routine. My life will have no meaning if I have to ditch my sweet treats too. I just won't read anything else about the harmful chemicals in processed food and then I can pretend it's perfectly safe to keep eating all of my favorite treats. Problem solved."

Only, the problem wasn't solved at all. The truth is, that during my weekly run to the supermarket, I paid more attention to which processed food products I could score a coupon deal on than to the ingredients used to make them.

If I was going to stick to my plan to improve my chronic illness symptoms, I couldn't ignore the fact that potentially harmful chemical ingredients are used to manufacture processed food. The more I read, the more I recognized that what I had been eating had compromised my health. After I discovered how many harmful chemical ingredients are used to make highly processed food and calculated the huge amounts of processed food I had ingested over the decades, I wasn't surprised that I was sick. I was surprised that I was still alive.

I exposed myself to a multitude of toxic ingredients every day through the food I chose to put into my body. Highly processed food is full of dyes, preservatives, trans fats, high fructose corn syrup, and a host of other manmade substances that our bodies were not designed to consume.[24]

Want an eye opener? Go grab a loaf of bread and take a look at the ingredients list. Then look for bread recipes online. Bread you make yourself requires flour, salt, yeast, a little sugar, and milk or water. Commercially produced bread contains dozens of ingredients including a whole lot of chemical additives.

When I began paying attention to the ingredient labels on packages, cans, and bottles, I knew a huge learning curve loomed ahead. It was obvious that I was going to have to change how I looked at food and learn to eat in a whole new way.

This is a partial list of potentially harmful ingredients found on highly processed food packaging labels.

- Artificial sweeteners, including aspartame and saccharine
- BHA and BHT preservatives and other substances that say added to preserve freshness

- Artificial food dyes and coloring. The petroleum-based dyes used in our country have been declared unsafe for use in foods in Europe.
- Artificial flavoring
- Nitrites, nitrates, and sulfites
- MSG (monosodium glutamate) Natural flavor is often a code word for MSG
- High fructose corn syrup
- Any chemical that says it is used as a food stabilizer
- Trans fats found in hydrogenated and partially hydro- genated oils

Any food that is prepackaged, processed beyond its natural state, and arrives at your local supermarket in a box, bottle, or can is quite likely to contain harmful ingredients. Some of the most problematic foods include:

- Sodas. These concoctions are little more than chemicals in a can or bottle.
- Lunchmeat, bacon, hot dogs. They are full of chemicals, dyes, and nitrites.
- Packaged cookies and candies. They are full of dyes, pre- servatives, shelf stabilizers, additives, and high fructose corn syrup.
- Artificial sweetener. It is not a natural substance.

All of these ingredients have been linked to a wide variety of chronic illnesses. I realized that if I wanted to improve my health, I had to stop eating so much processed food. I knew I would have to do the same thing I had done with exchanging harmful household products for safer ones. I would need to go slowly, not attempt to change too many things at once, and look for practical substitutes.

I took inventory of what was currently in my pantry and refrig- erator, read the labels on every food item in my home, and threw away everything that had harmful chemicals in it. This took time. I didn't check every item in a single day. I spent weeks reading the ingredients labels on my current food supply. I gradually replaced all the highly processed food I had been consuming with real foods like fruits, nuts, vegetables, grains, and seeds.

My first trip to the supermarket after my reality check about processed food was quite an adventure. I made a relatively short shopping list and planned a trip to the grocery store on a day I knew I didn't have to rush. I stopped in the produce section first to see what fresh fruits and vegetables were available at my local supermarket. I read every ingredient label on every item on my grocery list. I had jotted down the names of the most common toxic ingredients on an index card. If a product contained one or more of the harmful ingredients on my toxic list, I put that item back on the shelf. If I saw an ingredient name on a label that I didn't recognize, I looked it up on my smartphone. I typed, "Is (name of ingredient) harmful?" into my search engine about a million times during that first grocery store outing. Well, maybe, not a million, but it surely seemed like it when I was trying to figure out which food products were safe for me to eat. Because of the ever-increasing interest in eating healthy, there are a lot of smartphone apps to use to check food ingredients. Some cost a few dollars and others are free. I like the Fooducate app that lets you check the relative health of any food by scanning the barcode. It gives each product you scan a letter grade and additional health information about that food.

It was not practical to try to eliminate all packaged food in one fell swoop. It was a daunting task to change everything I currently ate to something that was healthier. I took my time and made only a few changes each week. I educated myself, read labels, and kept only those things in packages that have the fewest additives. I made a few changes at a time. Taking small steps helped me not feel so overwhelmed.

Consumers are becoming more aware of the harm processed food can cause and the big food companies are taking notice. When I first started changing the way I eat, it was difficult to find any packaged foods free of harmful additives unless I shopped at a health food store. Now I can find products with fewer chemicals at my local supermarket.

Even though I know processed food is not the healthiest choice, the practical reality is that sometimes I still eat it. There are occasions when it is impossible to access an exact ingredients list, such as eating in a restaurant, having dinner at a friend's house, or potluck dinners at church. I use two strategies to deal with the unknown.

- I plan ahead when possible. I check restaurant websites before eating out. Many include menus with ingredients listed for each item available. I find a meal with the fewest added chemicals and know what I'm going to order before I arrive.
- When it's not possible to plan ahead, I choose the healthiest options available. It's pretty obvious that salad, vegetables, and fruit will probably have less processed ingredients than a bag of packaged cookies or a casserole with multiple unknown ingredients.

Sometimes, I intentionally choose to eat processed food. My rule of thumb is that I eat only those items that have five ingredients or less listed on the label. Packaged items made with just a few ingredients are usually less processed and contain fewer additives than packaged foods with a long list of ingredients. I avoid items that contain the most harmful additives such as high fructose corn syrup, artificial dyes, preservatives, and other potentially harmful chemicals.

Here are a few examples:

- I occasionally eat potato chips, I choose the single serving size because, let's face it, once the bag is open, no matter how big that bag is, it becomes a single serving. I pick a brand that has only three ingredients: potatoes, salt, and oil rather than a brand that also contains added chemicals.

- I eat canned vegetables, beans, and legumes that contain no added ingredients. Beans are a good example of healthy canned items to keep on hand. I choose a brand that contains one ingredient: the beans. Canned beans are one of the few foods that are just as healthy canned as they are in the fresh version, as long as the beans do not contain added flavors, dyes, and preservatives. I keep my pantry stocked with black beans, pinto beans, red beans, and kidney beans which all contain high levels of good nutrients.
- I buy frozen fruit that contains only one ingredient, the fruit itself. Frozen fruit with no additives usually has as many nutrients as fresh fruit. This is a convenient food to keep on hand for the times a particular fresh fruit is out of season or I don't have time to run to the supermarket to buy fresh fruit. Bonus: frozen fruit makes delicious smoothies.
- I still use bottled condiments. Some folks make homemade everything. I'm not one of them. I can't see myself making mustard and ketchup.
- I eat a few types of cereal out of a box. I choose brands that contain the fewest chemical additives and the most natural ingredients. I also make homemade granola every now and then. You can find the recipe in Appendix II.
- I eat packaged yogurt. I choose Greek yogurt with no added ingredients or added sugar. Greek yogurt has fewer carbs and twice as much protein as regular yogurt.

I'm on a mission to create chemical-free strategies for healthy living, but I'm also determined to make my lifestyle practical. I don't have the time or the inclination to make every single thing I put into my mouth. So, I buy organic versions of food products when I can find them, I search for brands with the fewest chemicals, and I eat processed food only occasionally.

The first few months I was trying to improve my fibromyalgia symptoms, I stuck to eating real food 100% of the time. These days, my goal is to eat real food 90% of the time. It's liberating to know I can eat whatever I want with the remaining 10%. I recently took my grandchildren to their favorite bakery and chose a cookie for myself while they were debating the merits of the various goodies behind the glass display case. One bakery cookie wasn't going to derail my eating plan. Consuming an entire bag of processed cookies full of chemicals would.

My body confirmed that eliminating most processed foods from my diet was a good strategy for improving my fibromyalgia symptoms. On a scale of one to ten, my average pain level had dropped to around five after I replaced toxic household products and personal care items full of chemicals with safer options. After I eliminated most processed food from my diet, my average pain level dropped from five down to two or three most days. I had occasional spiking flares of increased pain, but these were becoming less frequent with each passing day. My chronic fatigue level had not decreased with the previous changes I made. However, after I eliminated most processed food from my diet, on a scale of one to ten, my fatigue level tumbled from a constant ten to hovering between five and eight.

Creating a chemical-free life was creating positive changes in my fibromyalgia symptom pattern. I was highly motivated to continue my personal research project. So, I munched on a handful of raw almonds as I considered additional lifestyle changes that held the potential to move me toward a healthier reality.

Dr. Norman Drops By

"Never eat anything that comes out of a box." These were the first words spoken by Dr. Richard C. Shelton, a visiting professor presenting a guest lecture at the medical school where I was on the faculty. Dr. Shelton teaches in the Psychiatry Department and does research on the links between nutrition, obesity, and depression as a member of the faculty at the University of Alabama in Birmingham School of Medicine. His topic was the origin of inflammation in the body and the effects of this inflammation on the nervous system. He commented that depression and fibromyalgia were two of the most common diseases to result from this inflammation.

Because Kathy's fibromyalgia was in the early stages of improvement from eliminating chemicals from her environment and making dietary changes, I was very interested in what Dr. Shelton had to share that day. He used detailed biochemical formulas to explain how the chemicals added to our food result in severe inflammation in our visceral fat, which is fatty tissue that surrounds the internal organs in the abdomen.[25] This was especially interesting to me because Kathy had recently read an article on the harm caused to our bodies by the buildup of visceral fat due to inflammation. One of the most harmful things about eating processed food is that consuming it increases visceral fat and visceral fat increases inflammation which influences the onset of many diseases.

Visceral fat is fat that you cannot see that wraps itself around your internal organs, especially organs in the digestive tract including the stomach, liver, and spleen. This type of fat causes chronic inflammation on a cellular level that leads to a host of diseases including fibromyalgia. It also contributes to aging, heart disease, diabetes, depression, sleep apnea, some types of cancer, dementia, and many other illnesses.

Eating processed food full of high fructose corn syrup, dyes, trans fats, and preservatives is one of the main triggers for developing visceral fat and the subsequent inflammation it causes. People who eat a lot of processed food, drink a lot of soda, and consume packaged products each day have high levels of visceral fat even if they are not visibly overweight.

It is interesting that visceral fat and inflammation are caused by our immune system reacting to the artificial chemicals found in processed food. Normally the immune reaction is triggered by a foreign substance in the body such as a disease-causing bacteria or virus which the immune system is designed to attack and destroy. For example, if you contract the flu, your body's immune system goes on high alert and swings into action to attack the flu virus. The immune system reacts with inflammation that causes fever, aches, pain, and fatigue which continue until the immune system does its job and eliminates the flu virus from your body. The inflammation and the symptoms resolve after the immune system has done its work.

When you consume the chemicals that are in processed food, the immune system springs into action as if it were attacking an unwanted invader like the flu. However, the inflammation created continues indefinitely. The preservatives, dyes, and other artificial ingredients added to processed foods are not substances that are found in nature. These chemicals are foreign to the body which has no way to metabolize them and excrete them. The body views these chemicals as an unwanted intruder it needs to destroy. So, the immune system incessantly attacks the patient's own body which results in a continuous inflammatory response.

This inflammation damages the body's own tissues. It releases increasing amounts of the normally helpful immune system chemicals into various parts of the body. This especially affects the nervous system which creates an unending loop of chronic pain and fatigue in response to the presence of chronic inflammation.

Artificial sweetener is one example of a substance that is not found in nature that is added to some types of processed food such as diet soda. When you drink a diet soda, it tastes sweet; but the body's metabolism does not recognize the artificial sweetener. This not only produces an inflammatory response;

it also can cause the body to gain weight by seeking real sugar to satisfy the internal sweet signal triggered by the artificial sweetener. Drinking both diet and regular soda has been linked to an increased risk of diabetes, hypertension, gout, elevated cholesterol levels, heart disease, and strokes.

High fructose corn syrup (HFCS) is another common additive in processed food. HFCS was initially developed in the late 1930s but it was not until the 1980s that HFCS was first added in significant amounts to processed food. In our country, there is a direct correlation from the 1980s to the present day between the increased rates of obesity and diabetes and the increased use of high fructose corn syrup in processed food. HFCS is seven times sweeter than natural sugar. It is very habit forming, especially in combination with salt and fat. The more you eat food with HFCS, the more you crave this type of processed food. And the inflammation rates in your body go up with every bite you swallow.

Trans fats are another common food additive. Fat molecules exist in both a *cis* and *trans* form. The liver is designed to process cis fat molecules. It is not designed to process trans fat molecules. This causes the trans fat molecules to build up in our systems which results in increased visceral fat and continuous inflammation. A splinter left under the skin indefinitely causes constant inflammation, pain, and swelling. The trans version of fat says inside the body indefinitely and causes a similar inflammatory response in the cells and organs inside the body.

The next time you are at the supermarket, look at the ingredients label on each of the packaged processed foods you are considering adding to your grocery cart. How many of them contain high fructose corn syrup, artificial sweetener, preservatives, dyes, and other unnatural chemicals? It doesn't take long to understand why Dr. Shelton said, "Never eat anything that comes out of a box."

Your Turn

1. Stop drinking soda. Whether you call it soda, pop, or soft drinks, it is nothing more than chemicals in a can, has absolutely no nutritional value, and has been shown to be detrimental to our overall health in numerous studies. My initial plan was to try to cut back on the number of sodas I drank each day, but that didn't work out very well, so I stopped drinking soda cold turkey. It was difficult the first couple of weeks which only confirmed how addicted I was to the stuff. I had headaches, anxiety, and obsessive cravings for a soda fix. After I got past the first two weeks of withdrawal symptoms, I didn't miss it at all. Write down how many cans of soda you currently drink per week. Create a plan for eliminating soda from your diet and write down the steps you plan to take to accomplish this.

2. Read the ingredients labels on any prepackaged items on your pantry shelves: cereal, cookies, candy, crackers, condiments, etc. Put everything that contains any of these harmful ingredients on the countertop: high fructose corn syrup (HFCS), trans fat, BHA or BHT preservatives, artificial colors, artificial flavors, artificial sweetener, monosodium glutamate (MSG). This will give you a clear picture of how many potentially harmful chemicals you currently consume. Identify the three items in your stack that contain the greatest number of toxic ingredients and toss them in the trash. Write down the number of processed food items you found that contain harmful chemicals. Write down the three items you plan to eliminate, the harmful chemicals that you found on the ingredient label of each item, and the date that you toss each one into the trash.

3. Choose three prepackaged items from your refrigerator/ freezer and read the ingredients labels. Find out what is used to make the frozen pizza, canned biscuits, hot dogs, and other processed food items you have stashed in the fridge. Look for homemade recipes in your favorite cookbook or online to replace at least one of the items. Plan a day this week to make it. Write down what you plan to make and add the date when you make it. Write down each of the three items you plan to eliminate, the harmful chemicals that you found on the ingredient label of each item, and the date that you toss each one into the trash.

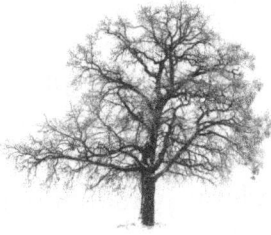

Priority 9: Make Smart Real Food Choices

I LOVED SCHOOL ART projects when I was a little girl. One year our teacher covered an entire wall of our room in white butcher paper and instructed us to draw pictures of things that grew from the earth that were good to eat. I used every color in the crayon box to fill my section of the mural with all kinds of fruits, vegetables, seeds, nuts, grains, and other real whole foods. I was proud of our class as I gazed at a wall full of beautiful food springing up from the ground, sprouting on bushes, and hanging from tree branches.

Somewhere between childhood and adulthood I lost my sense of wonder at the beauty of real food. I forgot that our bodies are designed with the ability to break down these natural foods to use for energy, growth, ramping up our immune system, and staying healthy. By the time I was diagnosed with fibromyalgia, I was eating way too many artificial food-like substances produced by multinational food conglomerates and not nearly enough of the real foods produced by nature.

Our relationship with food is complex. It is influenced by where we live, eating patterns we developed during childhood, food traditions we share with friends and extended family, our likes and dislikes, and our personal perceptions of what is healthy and what is unhealthy.

If you grew up in a family that emphasized healthy food choices, live in a part of the country replete with farmer's markets and health food stores, have easy access to a lot of fresh healthy foods, and are accustomed to swapping the latest organic vegetarian recipes with your friends, then you probably are already making wise choices regarding what you put into your body.

I grew up in the south where church potluck dinners are laden with casseroles full of processed ingredients, a vegetable plate at the local diner consists of four different carbohydrates plus a roll or cornbread, and any type of soda is considered a perfectly acceptable breakfast beverage. I had a tremendous learning curve to negotiate.

When I stopped eating processed foods that are full of potentially harmful chemical additives, I replaced them with a wide variety of whole real foods. I focused on foods full of antioxidants that boost the immune system and foods full of anti-inflammatory nutrients to help reduce the widespread excessive inflammation associated with fibromyalgia pain. If you want to see how eating real food can positively impact your health and reduce your fibromyalgia symptoms, there are some specific steps you can take.

Eat Foods That Contain Anti-inflammatory Nutrients

Since increased inflammation has been linked to so many health issues, I make sure I eat plenty of real foods loaded with anti-inflammatory nutrients. This helped reduce the inflammation in my body, decrease my pain level, and eventually changed my life in a way I never anticipated. There are many foods that reduce inflammation. These are 15 of my favorites. They are easy to find, simple to add to recipes, and most of them can be eaten raw or cooked.

- Almonds
- Cabbage
- Carrots
- Cauliflower
- Celery
- Cherries
- Honey. Raw local honey is the healthiest option.
- Lemons
- Limes
- Onions. Deep red and purple onions have more nutrients than white ones.
- Red radishes
- Spinach
- Squash
- Sweet potatoes. Eat them instead of white potatoes.
- Tomatoes
- Zucchini

There are also many herbs and spices that contain anti-inflammatory nutrients. They are easy to incorporate into many dishes. These are eight of my favorites:

- Basil
- Cayenne pepper
- Cilantro
- Cumin
- Garlic – fresh
- Ginger – fresh
- Oregano
- Turmeric

It is relatively simple to grow fresh basil, cilantro, and oregano. You can make your own herb garden with minimal equipment. All you need is seeds or small starter plants, potting soil, and a few empty containers. In the spring I plant pots of basil, parsley, cilantro, and rosemary on the deck just outside my kitchen door. Herbs can also be grown in small pots indoors if you have a place that gets adequate natural light. If you don't have a suitable space to grow your own herbs, you can buy fresh herbs or dried and ground herbs at your favorite supermarket.

It is easy to add foods rich in anti-inflammatory nutrients to your daily diet. I add herbs and spices to all my favorite recipes, sprinkle nuts and dried fruit over Greek yogurt, use dried cherries and almonds as a topping for granola, and add chopped garlic and onions to soups, spaghetti sauce, meat, poultry, vegetables, and just about everything I cook. You can find recipes that use foods and spices with anti-inflammatory nutrients in Appendix II.

Eat Foods Rich in Antioxidants

Foods that contain antioxidants are beneficial for revving up our immune systems. If you google the terms *antioxidant foods* or *super foods*, a whole lot of different lists will pop up. There are many delicious options. These are 15 of my favorite antioxidant rich foods. Four of these foods are on both my antioxidant and anti-inflammatory list: almonds, carrots, sweet potatoes, and tomatoes. I love eating real foods that have both since I double the health benefits with every bite.

- Almonds - plain with no salt
- Apples - try to find organic ones
- Beans - especially black and dark red
- Berries – blueberries and strawberries are my favorites
- Broccoli – steamed or roasted is delicious and nutritious. Add raw broccoli to salads.
- Carrots - eat them raw in salads or cooked as a side dish
- Grapes – dark red and dark purple
- Green and red peppers - try them in fajitas
- Oranges – choose whole fruit instead of juice

- Raisins - eat by the handful
- Sweet Potatoes – choose them more often than white potatoes
- Tea, green or black - drink several cups a day
- Tomatoes - very versatile raw or cooked
- Walnuts - sprinkle on cereal and yogurt
- Yogurt - Greek yogurt has more protein than regular yogurt

If you have trouble remembering all the different foods on these lists, just think colorfully. Usually the foods with the deepest colors have the most antioxidants. Here are a few examples.

- Blue: Blueberries
- Green: Broccoli, cabbage, kale, pears
- Orange: Carrots, pumpkin, sweet potatoes
- Red: Beets, red kidney beans, raspberries
- Purple: Blackberries, purple cabbage, plums
- Yellow: Chickpeas, pineapple, squash

Buy the Healthiest Real Food Available
The food lists above are just to give you a place to start. You can do your own research and discover your own favorites along the way. Here are a few ideas for buying the best real food you can find.

- Don't feel like you have to do everything at once. Add one new real food a day or one new food a week. Do whatever works best for you and your family. The important thing is to get started.
- Even fresh produce may contain chemical residue from pesticides and preservatives if it is commercially grown and shipped. When you buy fresh food from the supermarket you can remove some of the chemical residue by soaking the food in a vinegar and water solution. I've seen lots of variations of the water/vinegar soak. This one works best for me. Put ¼ cup of white vinegar in a

large glass or metal bowl. Don't use a plastic container because the vinegar may leach harmful substances from certain types of plastic into your food. Add fresh fruits and vegetables you buy at the supermarket like grapes, strawberries, apples, lemons, and tomatoes. Fill the container with enough water to completely cover the produce. Leave the produce submerged in this solution for fifteen minutes. Then rinse everything well with cold water and place in a colander to drain completely. This not only removes some of the chemical residue, it also helps the produce stay fresh for a longer period of time.[26]

- Buy fresh fruit and vegetables from local farmer's markets or directly from organic farmers. If the only practical option for you is the supermarket, buy organically certified produce when possible. Talk to the produce manager at your grocery store to see if he purchases any local fruits and vegetables. Locally grown produce may have some pesticide residue depending on the growing methods used by the farmer, but it is rarely sprayed with the extra layer of chemicals to preserve freshness that is often added to produce that is shipped long distances.

- Look for someone in your area that raises organically certified chickens and range fed organic beef. Animals that have not been given antibiotics and hormones are less toxic because they are raised using natural methods.

- Find the best places to shop for real food in your area. You can find organic chicken, beef, and all kinds of organic produce at organic grocery store chains like Earth Fare and Whole Foods Markets. You can find some organic chemical-free meat and produce at big box stores like Walmart, Target, and Costco. Safeway grocery stores have a brand called O Organic. The label looks the same no matter which department you are in so it is easy to spot the organic items on the shelves. A word of caution here. Just because a product has an organic label, that doesn't mean it is guaranteed to be free of harmful additives. Always read the ingredients label on any prepackaged manufactured food product before you toss it into your shopping cart so that you know exactly what is in it.

- Buy eggs that come from free range chickens that have not been given antibiotics and hormones. I buy local eggs from a friend who raises free range chickens. The yolks are a much deeper yellow than commercially produced eggs you find at most supermarkets. The eggs have a much richer and satisfying flavor than the ones from the store. And they are free of chemicals. Some folks are skittish about buying eggs that come straight from the chicken because they have no expiration date stamped on them and there might be a feather or two stuck to the shells. Consider this: eggs you buy from the grocery store may be several weeks old before they are put into the carton, date stamped, and shipped. I learned a great trick for testing the freshness of eggs from fellow missionaries when we lived in Colombia that I still use to this day. Put the eggs you plan to use in the bottom of a deep bowl with enough room for each egg to lay flat on its side at the bottom of the bowl. Fill the bowl with enough cold water to cover the eggs by three or four inches. If the eggs stay flat with their sides still touching the bottom of the bowl, they are very fresh. You can use them for scrambling, frying, baking, or whatever you want. If any of the eggs turn so that they are standing up on end with one of the points still securely resting on the bottom of the bowl, it's not quite as fresh. Those eggs are fine to use for baking, but they are a little too old to use for scrambling and other quickly cooked dishes. If an egg floats away from the bottom of the bowl toward the top of the water with no part of the egg resting on the bottom of the bowl, it is past its prime and may contain harmful bacteria. Throw those eggs away.

Aim for the 90%-10% Goal

I discovered early on that it was not practical for me to eat real food 100% of the time. I aim for the 90%-10% goal. I eat real food free of chemicals and preservatives most of the time. Some days this just isn't feasible. I'm running errands and have to grab a quick meal on the go that includes some processed food with harmful additives. I'm invited to dinner at a friend's house. I have no way of knowing all the ingredients used to prepare the food. My goal is to eat real food at least 90% of the time. Because there are a thousand ways that real life gets in the way, despite my best intentions, having a 10% flexibility option built into each day makes it easier for me to consistently stick to my healthy eating plan the other 90 % of the time.

Use an Elimination Diet to Check for Food Allergies and Sensitivities

One more food issue I had to deal with was investigating the possibility that I might have one or more food sensitivities or food allergies. Food sensitivities are not quite as severe as a true food allergy, but any type of food intolerance can be harmful to your body.

People can be allergic to almost any food but there are eight primary groups that cause the most common food allergies and food sensitivities: shellfish, gluten, dairy, soy, peanuts, fish, eggs, and tree nuts (walnuts, almonds, cashews, etc.).

I was already allergic to shellfish so I had stopped eating it long before I created a healthy living plan to cope with my fibromyalgia symptoms. After I completed an elimination diet, I discovered I also had food intolerances and sensitivities to dairy and peanuts that increased my fibromyalgia symptoms. Vic will explain how to do an elimination diet when he drops by later on in this chapter.

If you have a food allergy or intolerance, there are many delicious and nutritious substitutes to replace the types of food you need to avoid. I don't have a problem with any nuts other than peanuts. I stopped eating peanuts and peanut butter. I eat tree nuts and almond butter instead. There are other flavorful nut butters to try like cashew butter. If you are allergic to all nuts, you may want to try sunflower butter made from sunflower seeds.

I discovered I also have a food sensitivity to dairy products. I'm a huge fan of ice cream. I love cheese on just about anything. But I am a bigger fan of feeling better and staying healthy. I eliminated most dairy products from my diet.

I use almond milk instead of cow's milk. Other options are coconut milk, rice milk, soy milk, and cashew milk. I can eat things cooked with a small amount of milk as long as milk is not the primary ingredient. I eat a single serving of Greek yogurt once or twice a week without difficulty. I do not drink cow's milk and I no longer eat ice cream. I feel so much better that I haven't even missed it. And the truth is that I probably already had eaten enough ice cream in the past five decades to last an entire lifetime. (Hope note. Seven years after detoxifying my body, I now am able to eat some dairy foods occasionally without any adverse effects. I occasionally eat soft cheeses like mozzarella but avoid hard cheeses like cheddar.)

Make Real Food More Convenient

Processed food is not healthy, but it is convenient. So, I looked for ways to make real food convenient too. Here are a few ideas.

- Make your own sandwich meat. Instead of buying processed lunchmeat full of nitrates and nitrites, prepare your own meat for sandwiches, put individual servings in freezer safe containers, and take out what you need as you need it. I grill chicken in large batches and freeze it so that I have it available to make a grilled chicken sandwich, fajitas, or a grilled chicken salad. I cook a large roast in the crockpot, divide it into individual portion sizes and pop them into the freezer so that preparing a roast beef sandwich is a snap.

- Create homemade frozen dinners. I always cook more servings than I need for a meal and freeze part of it for future use. Here are a few suggestions. Make enough chicken stir fried rice for two meals instead of just the one you are planning to eat that night and freeze the extra one for a future meal. Make a huge pot of soup or stew and freeze part of it. I freeze some of the extra food I cook in family size batches. I freeze some in single serving portions for those days when I need to grab a quick meal just for myself.
- Cook your own sweet treats. Love sweet stuff? I gave up processed packaged cookies and candies. But I still enjoy sweet treats that I make myself from real food ingredients like whole wheat flour, organic raw sugar, local raw honey, molasses, oatmeal, dried fruit, ground flaxseed, and nuts.
- Produce homemade snack foods. Need more ideas? Freeze grapes and fresh pineapple and eat them frozen for a quick, cool refreshing treat. Prefer salty treats? Buy almonds and walnuts in bulk when you find them on sale and store in airtight containers in your pantry. Add chopped nuts to recipes or eat whole raw nuts by the handful for a crunchy satisfying snack. Make your own microwave popcorn using organic popcorn kernels. You can find the recipe in Appendix II.
- Bake your own bread. We love homemade bread for breakfast. I make quick breads like muffins and scones. I freeze them and then just take them out one at a time as needed.

Heat each serving for 45 seconds in the microwave. If you like pancakes and waffles, you can make them in large batches to freeze and you have a healthier version than the commercially produced frozen ones in a box which often contain harmful additives. Check out Appendix II for ideas and recipes for preparing your own healthy foods from scratch.

I'm not going to gloss over reality here. Cooking whole foods from scratch will take extra planning and preparation time. Just remember you don't have to do everything at once. You can make your own convenience foods a little at a time. Pace yourself. Every positive step you take is one small step toward creating a healthier life.

The more real food I ate, the better I felt. Implementing the previous practical priorities decreased my pain level from ten to an average of between three to five. After I eliminated most processed food from my diet and replaced it with real foods rich in antioxidants and anti-inflammatory nutrients, something amazing happened. Although I still had severe chronic fatigue, occasional spiking pain flares, and moderate pain in my knees and legs, the average daily pain level in the rest of my muscles and joints tumbled down to zero.

Dr. Norman Drops By

Hippocrates, the famous Greek physician who is often considered to be the father of western medicine, said, "Let food be thy medicine and medicine be thy food." That is still good advice. The food we put into our bodies either causes disease or promotes health. Think about these three things as you implement strategies to eat the best real food possible.

Antioxidants Boost the Immune System

Eating foods that contain antioxidants is a smart choice for anyone because antioxidants boost the immune system, keep us healthy, and can help us recover when we are sick. Antioxidants are chemical compounds that prevent the process known as oxidation in which oxygen combines with another chemical causing destructive results. A familiar example of the oxidation process can be seen when iron is exposed to oxygen resulting in rust. Most of us have observed how corrosive rust can be to metallic objects.

In our bodies the rust equivalent is known as free radicals. They are as destructive to our cells and organs as rust is to metal. Free radicals form in our bodies when we breathe air that is polluted by chemicals from industrial waste, cigarette smoke, cleaning products, products that contain fragrance, and other environmental chemicals. If you eat a lot of highly processed food that is loaded with chemical ingredients, then the level of free radicals in your body increases. This causes constant damage to your body. The free radicals combine with tissue in the body which results in inflammation and destruction to the cells. It is as if you are corroding all your organs and internal systems with rust.

Fortunately, there are many foods which are loaded with antioxidants. The antioxidants found in foods are a natural wonder. They not only help prevent destruction to our cells from free radicals, they also help repair damage that is already there. Foods loaded with antioxidants help prevent disease and boost our immune systems. They effectively combine with the free radicals before the free radicals can oxidize the body's cells and tissues causing damage and inflammation. The antioxidants neutralize the free radicals and the inflammation is canceled out.

While research is ongoing, there is a great deal of anecdotal evidence that foods rich in antioxidants promote health and well-being. I have seen this with my own wife. The more food rich in antioxidants and anti-inflammatory nutrients that Kathy ate, the more her health improved. And because I was eating the same thing, so did mine.

Anti-inflammatory Foods Reduce Pain

Researchers may disagree about many things concerning fibromyalgia. But one thing is clear: people who suffer from fibromyalgia have a lot of inflammation in their bodies. Chronic inflammation also appears to play a role in the onset of autoimmune disorders like rheumatoid arthritis, lupus, and polymyalgia rheumatica, as well as diseases such as asthma, ulcerative colitis, and Crohn's disease. Research is being done on the possible link between chronic inflammation and cardiovascular disease and the possibility that it is a factor in some types of cancer. Eating processed food that is full of harmful chemicals and synthetic additives increases the inflammation in your body and inflammation increases pain levels. Eating a wide variety of wholesome real food full of anti-inflammatory nutrients reduces both inflammation and pain. Choose options from the lists Kathy shares in this chapter to add foods to your diet that contain both antioxidants and anti-inflammatory nutrients.

Complete an Elimination Diet to Check for Food Allergies, Intolerances, and Sensitivities

If you have been diagnosed with fibromyalgia or any type of chronic illness, have vague symptoms that don't match any disease pattern, or just don't feel quite up to par, you may have some type of food allergy or food intolerance. I recommend consulting your family physician or an allergist to get more information about food allergies, food intolerances, and food sensitivities. It is important to talk to your doctor before starting any food modification plan. After you have discussed this with your physician, you can try the elimination diet at home to test for food intolerances.

People can be allergic to almost any food but there are eight primary food groups that cause the most common food allergies and food sensitivities: shellfish, gluten, dairy, soy, peanuts, fish, eggs, and tree nuts (walnuts, almonds, cashews, etc.).

You need to eliminate all of these foods temporarily in order to evaluate whether or not you have a food intolerance to any of them. Here's a step by step guide to completing an elimination diet.

- For one month, stop eating all shellfish, gluten, dairy products, soy, peanuts, fish, eggs, and tree nuts. It will take about a month to get these foods out of your system. It is important to completely eliminate all eight groups so that you can properly test for food allergies, intolerances, and sensitivities.

- After one month, start eating shellfish again. Do not add back any foods from the other food groups. Eat some type of shellfish every day for one week. At the end of the week evaluate how you feel. Do you feel worse than you did when you were not eating shellfish? Do you have any increase in symptoms such as pain, fatigue, headache, digestive distress, or general malaise? If you have any of these symptoms, you may have a sensitivity or intolerance to shellfish that is contributing to your fibromyalgia pain. Do not eat any more shellfish and consult your physician. If you develop severe symptoms while eating shellfish such as breaking out in hives, swelling of the lips or tongue, constriction in the throat, chest pressure, or difficulty breathing, this may indicate you have a true food allergy. Stop eating shellfish immediately and consult your physician. If the increased symptoms are extreme go to the nearest emergency medical facility. This type of severe response may indicate the onset of anaphylactic shock which is a life-threatening condition that requires immediate medical attention.

- If you had increased symptoms to shellfish, you will have to get the shellfish out of your system before checking any of the other food groups. Wait one week before testing another food. If you noticed no difference when adding shellfish back to your diet, you can keep eating shellfish whenever you want, and you can add back one more food group to test for intolerance.

- You are ready to test another food group. Add foods that contain soy back to your diet. Eat something with soy in it every day for one week. Do not add back any foods from the other remaining food groups. At the end of the week evaluate how you feel. Do you feel worse than you did when you were not eating soy? Do you have any increase in symptoms such as pain, fatigue, headache, digestive distress, or general malaise? If you notice no difference when adding soy back to your diet, you can keep eating soy. However, if you have any increase in your symptoms, you may have a sensitivity or intolerance to soy that is contributing to your fibromyalgia pattern. Do not eat any more soy and consult your physician. If you develop severe symptoms while eating soy such as breaking out in hives, swelling of the lips or tongue, constriction in the throat, chest pressure, or difficulty breathing, this may indicate you have a true food allergy. Stop eating soy immediately and consult your physician. If the increased symptoms are extreme go to the nearest emergency medical facility. This type of response may indicate the onset of anaphylactic shock which is a life-threatening condition that requires immediate medical attention.

- If you noticed no difference when adding soy back to your diet, you can keep eating soy and you can add back one more food group to test for intolerance. If you noticed any kind of increased symptoms, stop eating soy and consult your physician. Wait one week before testing another food. You need to get the soy out of your system before checking any of the other food groups.

- You are ready to test another food group. Add foods that contain gluten back to your diet. Eat something with gluten in it every day for one week. Do not add back any foods from the other remaining food groups. At the end of the week evaluate how you feel. Do you feel worse than you did when you were not eating gluten? Do you have any increase in symptoms such as pain, fatigue, headache, digestive distress, or general malaise? If you notice no difference when adding gluten back to your diet, you can keep eating gluten. However, if you have any of these symptoms, you may have a sensitivity or intolerance to gluten that is contributing to your fibromyalgia pattern. Do not eat any more gluten and consult your physician. If you develop severe symptoms while eating gluten such as breaking out in hives, swelling of the lips or tongue, constriction in the throat, chest pressure, or difficulty breathing, this may indicate you have a true food allergy. Stop eating gluten immediately and consult your physician. If the increased symptoms are extreme go to the nearest emergency medical facility. This type of response may indicate the onset of anaphylactic shock which is a life-threatening condition that requires immediate medical attention.

- If you noticed no difference when adding gluten back to your diet, you can keep eating gluten and you can add back one more food group to test for intolerance. If you noticed any kind of increased symptoms, stop eating gluten and consult your physician. Wait one week before testing another food. You need to get the gluten out of your system before checking any of the other food groups.

Repeat these steps for the five remaining food groups: dairy, peanuts, fish, eggs, and tree nuts (walnuts, almonds, cashews, etc.). Add each group back one at time, evaluate your results, eliminate the food if it increases your symptoms, continue eating foods in that group if you notice no changes in your symptom pattern, and contact your physician as needed per the instructions given in the steps for the other food groups.

After you complete the elimination diet for these eight common food allergy triggers, evaluate whether any other food may be causing your fibromyalgia symptoms to increase. Keep a record for one month of everything you eat each day and make a note of the days your symptoms are the most severe so that you can evaluate if some specific food is making your symptoms worse. For example, if you notice that your symptoms seem to spike every time you eat bananas or that they are worse on the days you eat a food from the nightshade family such as tomatoes, repeat the elimination diet for that specific food or food group. If your symptoms improve greatly when leaving off this food or food group, try leaving it out of your diet for a month to see if your symptoms improve.

Discuss any food allergies or intolerances you discover while doing the elimination diet with your doctor. It is especially important to determine if you have a food intolerance or a true food allergy. Food intolerances can increase your symptom levels and cause discomfort. True food allergies can cause severe medical problems, including anaphylaxis which can result in death. You need to be under a physician's care if you have a true food allergy so that you can get prevention information and receive appropriate treatment recommendations.

Your Turn

1. Pick seven foods from the list of foods and spices that contain anti-inflammatory nutrients. Eat at least one of

these foods and use at least one of the spices every day for a week. List the foods and spices here and make a note of the day(s) you use each one. At the end of the week, put a checkmark by the foods and spices that you feel you can incorporate easily into your permanent eating plan.

2. To boost your immune system, choose at least one food from the list of foods that contain antioxidants to eat each day for a month. List the foods here and make a note of the day(s) you eat each one. At the end of the month, put a checkmark by the foods that you feel you can incorporate easily into your permanent eating plan.

3. Do the elimination diet to check for food allergies or sensitivities to the top eight potentially problematic food groups: shellfish, gluten, dairy, soy, peanuts, fish, eggs, and tree nuts (walnuts, almonds, cashews, etc.). Consult your family physician or an allergist if you have any type of reaction to a specific food or food group. List the date you start the elimination diet and the date that you add each of the eight food groups back. Put a circle around any of the food groups that seemed to cause an increase in your symptoms. List the specific symptoms you notice that appear to be associated with eating that particular food.

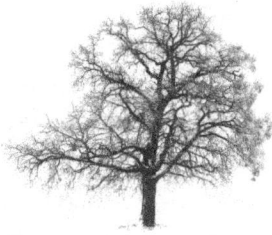

Priority 10: Move Every Day

AFTER I ELIMINATED products made with toxic chemicals from my home environment, stopped eating so much processed food, and consistently ate lots of real food with antioxidants and anti-inflammatory nutrients, I had fewer and fewer fibromyalgia pain flares. I had little to no pain at all in most of my muscles and joints. I still had pain in my legs and my knees and really aggravating chronic fatigue that often hindered my ability to function normally.

Restoration was occurring daily, not only physically, but also emotionally and spiritually. I was full of hope and focused on possibilities rather than problems. Initially, dealing with the ravages of fibromyalgia knocked my faith for a loop. I was still skittish and skeptical about faith issues. But, by this time in the process, I was finding encouragement from occasionally reading the Bible or a short devotional. These verses from the Old Testament book of Isaiah were especially meaningful: "He gives strength to the weary and increases the power of the weak. Even youths grow tired and weary, and young men stumble and fall; but those who hope in the Lord will renew their strength.

They will soar on wings like eagles; they will run and not grow weary, they will walk and not be faint." (Isaiah 40:29-31 NIV)

I love the poetic images in these words. Soaring on eagle's wings would be awesome. Who wouldn't want to fly? Running and not growing weary seemed like a spectacular impossibility since I was incapacitated by chronic fatigue. I was grateful for days that I managed simply to walk and not faint.

I reread these verses while I looked for additional ways to improve my health. I found multiple articles about the importance of exercise both for preventing disease and for coping with chronic illness. There were even specific suggestions that moving more might help reduce my fibromyalgia symptoms.

I didn't know whether to laugh or cry. It was quite comical to picture myself doing any kind of exercise since I still had horrible chronic fatigue symptoms. Most days just getting out of bed, struggling into my clothes, and creeping into the kitchen to prepare breakfast left me absolutely drained. How could I exercise when I was constantly exhausted? How could I move muscles and joints that had been inactive for ages? The pain was finally better. What if jostling around made it worse again?

As it turns out, all those voices encouraging me to get up and get moving were right.[27] I had become quite sedentary due to the fallout from my fibromyalgia symptoms. I hadn't used most of my muscles and joints in years. I had a lot of work to do to rebuild my stamina and retrain my muscles and joints to operate like they were designed to function.

If you love to walk, bike, hike, lift weights, swim, kayak, and run marathons, you can skip this chapter. If your idea of sufficient exercise is walking from the couch to the refrigerator to grab a snack, read on.

We all have different symptom patterns with chronic illness. You may need to modify the recommendations in this chapter to fit your specific situation. If you have any type of serious injury or physical condition that limits your ability to exercise, you will need to consider what is feasible for you. Consult your physician before starting any exercise program. If you do not have any current injuries and your doctor gives you the go ahead, here are six practical suggestions for adding movement to your daily routine.

Be Realistic

I'm not very athletic. But before I got sick, I could walk three miles a day, hike up a steep mountain, swim laps for thirty minutes at a time, chase my grandchildren around the park, and shop all day long. I had to admit that these might not be attainable goals for me now. Just because I couldn't do the things I used to do before, didn't mean I had to settle for doing nothing at all. Finding a realistic way to incorporate movement into my daily routine was essential.

Even if you are not ill, it is important to have pragmatic expectations about what you can realistically add to your day. You may have time considerations due to work and family responsibilities. Patience will be required if it has been years since you attempted any form of exercise or if exercise has never been a part of your life before.

Part of my personal reality check was knowing I needed to detoxify my body from chemical exposure and boost my immune system by eating lots of healthy real foods before I attempted adding any form of exercise to my daily routine. I had done that. I was ready for this next step.

Start Slowly

When I considered adding exercise back to my daily routine, I was dealing with constant chronic fatigue and other lingering fibromyalgia symptoms. I hadn't done any type of exercise at all in years. My muscles were atrophied and my joints were stiff from inactivity. I wanted to move but I wasn't sure that I could. Then I read about a suggestion for walking just one minute a day. That encouraged me so much. I thought that even in my weakened state I could manage to walk for one minute.

So, I walked around the inside of my house for one minute once a day for several weeks. After I got used to that, I started walking two minutes each day. I slowly added minutes until I was walking fifteen minutes at a time. I was strolling, not race walking, but I was up and going. It was a start.

When the weather was nice, I walked outside. Moving around in the sunshine is a great mood booster. I gradually added swimming, light weight lifting, tai chi, and a stretching regimen to my routine. Adding this small amount of movement and exercise to my day not only helped with my physical symptoms, it also elevated my mood.

Use a Step Counter

These days I use a step counter to keep track of how much I walk. I use a fitness tracker that I wear on my wrist. Options for counting steps include simple pedometers, activity trackers like Fitbit or Garmin VivoFit, and fitness apps on smartphones.

You can improve your health and stamina by slowly increasing the number of steps you normally take. Track how many steps you take each day for a week to get the starting number of how many steps you normally take during a day. Add 100 steps to your average. If your average number of steps per day is currently 1000, try walking 1100 steps each day until you feel comfortable with that and then add 100 more steps. It is the same principle as counting minutes. Start where you are and increase the amount you move very slowly over an extended period of time.

The average number of steps per day for a healthy adult is around 5000. If you have fibromyalgia, your average step count is probably much lower than that. Mine was only 1000 when I started. Some fitness experts recommend aiming for 10,000 steps a day to maximize the health benefits of walking.

That is not practical for someone with fibromyalgia, especially in the first stages of adding movement to your day. If you have a chronic illness, don't focus on any maximum recommended number. Start with your unique current average number of steps per day no matter what it is, be thankful that you are able to move at all, and celebrate every single increase you achieve.

Stretch

I know some folks who love yoga or similar programs. I am too uncoordinated to get the hang of contorting my body into all those odd positions. I do a ten-minute tai chi routine every morning and some simple arm, back, and leg stretches. Since I was being realistic, I started out by doing only two reps of each stretch and gradually worked up to twenty-five reps over a period of weeks.

There are books that describe exercise programs designed specifically for folks with a chronic illness or a sedentary lifestyle. Look on amazon.com or browse through your favorite bookstore. Ask your doctor for recommendations on simple stretching exercises that are appropriate for your current physical condition and age. Check out exercise routines for beginners on YouTube and other online sources.

I learned my first tai chi moves by following along with an eight-minute YouTube video by tai chi expert Don Fiori: 8 Minute Daily Tai Chi. Tai chi is an intentional movement and controlled breathing practice that originated in ancient China. It is especially suitable for people with fibromyalgia because it increases range of motion, strengthens muscles, and improves memory, flexibility, and balance through a series of low intensity flowing movements that don't put stress on muscles and joints.

Swim

Swimming is a great way to exercise your muscles and joints without putting weight bearing pressure and stress on them. I had access to a swimming pool for two years. I began by swimming to one end of the pool. I rested for a while and then swam back to the other end. That was all I could manage at first. Gradually I worked up to swimming laps for five minutes before I had to rest. Eventually, I was staying in the pool for thirty to forty-five minutes at a time several times a week. I swam laps part of the time and did leg lifts and stretches holding on to the side of the pool part of the time. I no longer have year-round access to a swimming pool so I have substituted walking for swimming. I still like to swim when there is a pool available.

Swimming is a great example of substituting one thing for another to fit your particular needs. If you have any type of injury that prevents you from walking, you may be able to swim without difficulty. If you don't have access to a pool, you may be able to use a stationary exercise bicycle which also puts less stress on bones and joints. With either choice, follow the same steps listed above. Start slowly and gradually increase the time you spend doing whichever exercise you choose.

Spend Time Outside
Having a chronic illness that limited my normal social interaction caused me to feel isolated and depressed. It lifts my spirits to get outside and walk a little even if it is only for a few minutes at a time. My husband and I love to go camping. When I was experiencing severe fibromyalgia symptoms, I didn't have the stamina to hike like we did before I became ill. There are other ways to enjoy the beauty of nature. You can stroll on a boardwalk at the beach, walk on a level path through the woods, or just go outside and saunter around the block near your home.

I have more energy and stamina now but I'm still not back to the activity level I enjoyed before I was diagnosed with fibromyalgia. I realize that years of inactivity caused my muscles to atrophy. I have added light weight lifting to my routine in an effort to increase my muscle strength and restore my stamina.

We have a weight machine at our house. I started out by using five-pound weights and then increased to ten-pound weights. I do one series of exercises on the weight machine to strengthen my arms and another series of exercises to strengthen my legs. If you do not have a weight machine at home, you can look into joining a gym. Some hospitals and medical facilities offer wellness programs that allow you to use their exercise equipment for a small monthly fee. Some of these facilities have a wellness program director that will help you design the best exercise routine for your needs. If that is not feasible, you can purchase small hand weights quite inexpensively at your nearest big box store.

Everyone reading this book will be at a different stage of health and energy level. Many readers may be dealing with fibromyalgia plus another chronic illness. The key is to do something, even if it is only getting up off the couch and walking through the rooms of your house for one minute each morning and afternoon.

I started the one-minute walking plan when I was still quite ill. I didn't add swimming, stretches, tai chi, and weights until some of my symptoms had resolved and I was starting to feel better.

I paced myself with exercise and with the other changes I made. Taking one step at a time, making one small change at a time, adding one new healthy food at a time, eliminating one chemical at a time did not seem as overwhelming as trying to do everything at once. Step by step, little by little, I found out that it is possible to gradually move toward recovery.

I still had pain in my legs and my knees and moderate to severe chronic fatigue. However, after adding movement to my day, I rarely had pain in my other muscles. The spiking pain flares completely disappeared. I may never get back to the level of physical activity I was able to enjoy before fibromyalgia, but I'm grateful for every single bit of improved mobility.

Dr. Norman Drops By

Exercise is beneficial in maintaining health. Exercise has been shown to improve heart disease, hypertension, diabetes, depression, fibromyalgia, and many other illnesses. A great deal of research is being done at this time to analyze the effects of exercise on improving health and moderating disease. For doctors and scientists, the primary questions regarding exercise are: Why does exercise help improve symptoms? Can exercise be harmful to patients? What is happening with the patient's body that causes this improvement in such a diverse assortment of illnesses?

The most recent research shows that there is a relationship between exercise and the levels of natural chemicals called cytokines in the body. There are two types of cytokines: good cytokines that decrease inflammation and bad cytokines that increase inflammation. The preliminary research conclusions show that the level of exercise determines the total levels of the good and bad cytokines as well as their ratio to one other.

With mild to moderate exercise, the total levels of good cytokines increase as well as show a relative boost to the levels of bad cytokines. If one goes past moderate exercise into strenuous exercise, the bad cytokines increase in total and relative levels resulting in increased inflammation that is harmful to the body.[28]

It is important to create an exercise plan that takes your personal current health status and age into consideration. The medical research to date concludes that mild to moderate exercise such as swimming, walking, riding an exercise bicycle, and tai chi are effective for raising the good cytokine levels and decreasing inflammation. The research suggests that strenuous exercise can actually be harmful for a patient dealing with a chronic inflammatory illness such as fibromyalgia. This means that you need to find your personal sweet spot for helpful exercise without overdoing it.

There are some specific exercise strategies for people who have a chronic illness. A patient who is severely limited in his or her mobility due to fibromyalgia, another chronic illness, or an injury can benefit from mild exercise. If all you are able to do is simply take a few steps inside your home, your good cytokine levels will improve with movement. Start where you are and do what you can. Try walking one minute through the rooms of your home every day. Or stroll around the block with a friend after dinner three times a week. Even this small step can be of great benefit to a patient working toward improving his or her fibromyalgia symptoms.

If you have fibromyalgia or another chronic illness and are ready to add movement to your daily routine, consult your physician to verify that you are healthy enough to exercise and get your doctor's recommendations for a plan tailored to meet your specific needs.

There are three practical strategies that can help you achieve your goals for adding movement to your day. Your exercise program needs to be planned, tailored to fit your unique situation, and it needs to be practical.

Plan Your Strategy
You need to start by deciding exactly what you would like to accomplish by adding movement to your daily routine. If your goal is to exercise more, you need to decide which exercise you want to do and how many times a week you will try to do this. Instead of making a vague general statement like, "I'm going to start some kind of exercise program sometime," create a more specific plan. For example, "I will walk five minutes a day, three times a week," or "I will swim three laps in the pool twice a week." Write your plan down and add when you plan to do each activity to your daily calendar. Put a checkmark by each activity when you complete it to verify that you have accomplished your goal.

Fit Your Plan to Your Fitness Level
It can be overwhelming to think of committing to something new long term. You need to fit your plan to your current fitness level. Have a specific beginning and ending time for your specific exercise strategy in mind before you even start. Write down the timeframe on your calendar. In the beginning, I suggest planning to implement your goal for just a few weeks and never for longer than one month. If one week is all you think you can manage, then pick the specific week you are going to implement your plan and write it down. After the initial goal is met, congratulate yourself that you completed your goal. Assess your fitness level after you complete your specific timeframe for the activity you have chosen. As your fitness level improves, you will be able to choose different types of activities and longer timeframes for doing them.

Plan a Goal That You Can Accomplish
If you are currently sedentary due to a chronic illness or because you haven't done any kind of exercise in years, it is not practical to start off by saying you will run three miles every day. However, it may be completely doable to decide you will walk around outside in the yard three days each week for the next three weeks. Make your beginning goal something small enough that you have a reasonable expectation that you will accomplish it. After you meet your first goal, set a new goal that is also small enough to reach. Keep doing this over time and you will ultimately reach a bigger goal than you had anticipated when you first started your new exercise plan.

Your Turn

1. Describe your current fitness level. Are you completely sedentary? Do you have fibromyalgia or some other limiting chronic illness? Are you reasonably healthy but want

to add more movement to your daily routine? What are your goals for adding movement to your day?

2. Pick one specific new activity to add to your day: walking, swimming, riding an exercise bicycle, stretching, weight lifting, using a step counter, tai chi, or another movement activity of your choice. Write down which exercise you plan to do, how many days a week you plan to do it, and how many minutes you plan to do it on the days you choose.

3. Put your exercise plan on your calendar. Include a beginning and ending date for completing the activity that you choose. Put a checkmark beside each day that you complete your written goal for that day. Put a star by the day you completed your plan. You did it! Decide what your next movement goal is and go for it.

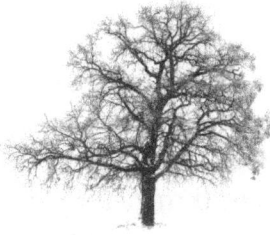

Priority 11: Get Enough Sleep

I NSOMNIA WAS AN unexpected and frustrating symptom of my fibromyalgia pattern. Before my chronic illness struck, I was an extremely sound sleeper. I have slept through tornados, blaring car alarms, and neighborhood Fourth of July fireworks shenanigans. When we were missionaries in Colombia, I slept through a bomb exploding in a house down the street. It blew out all the windows in the apartment building next to ours; but it didn't wake me up. So, it came as quite a shock to my system when I had difficulty falling asleep and staying asleep. My doctor prescribed a sleep medication. This helped me to catch a few fitful hours of sleep most nights; but I never felt rested when I woke up in the morning.

Sleep disturbances in fibromyalgia may be related to the disease process itself, as well as to the cellular damage that results from exposure to chemicals in our food and environment. I had chronic fatigue that was partly due to my particular fibromyalgia symptom pattern. The fact that I had not slept well during the three years I had been ill was also a contributing factor. My body had forgotten the natural rhythm of sleep.

By the time I decided to address my sleep issues, I had detoxified my body by creating a chemical-free life. I had stopped eating most processed food. I was eating a lot of real food full of antioxidants and anti-inflammatory nutrients to boost my immune system and decrease the inflammation in my body. I had added movement to my daily routine. My fibromyalgia symptoms had improved significantly. I still had pain in my legs and my knees and moderate to severe chronic fatigue. But I rarely had pain in my other muscles and joints, and the spiking pain flares, numbness and tingling in my extremities, fibro fog, dizziness, difficulty breathing, and balance issues had completely resolved.

I was thankful for this amazing level of improvement. Because I still had awful insomnia and persistent chronic fatigue symptoms, the next thing I investigated was ways to deal with my compromised sleep pattern.

As I roamed around cyberspace scrolling for information, everything I read about sleep issues indicated that I needed to reset my natural sleep cycle. Be sure to consult your physician before trying any plan that involves changing your present medications or taking supplements. Here's what I did.

I stopped taking prescription sleep medication.
This type of drug is intended for short-term use. It is not designed to be used for longer than a few days at a time and should never be used for more than a few weeks at a time. Sleep induced by medication does not follow a natural sleep cycle pattern. In addition to these factors, using a manufactured pharmaceutical for sleep defeated my goal of creating a chemical-free life because it added another chemical substance to my body on a daily basis. I had used prescription sleep medication for years, a far longer time than is normally recommended, in a desperate attempt to get whatever sleep I could manage.

I knew I needed to make a change so I dove into the deep end of the pool and stopped taking prescription sleep medication cold turkey. This was a nerve-racking endeavor. I had been taking my itty-bitty sleep helpers so long, I was psychologically dependent on them. Even though I knew it was an unwise choice for creating an effective long-term solution to my insomnia, it was my security blanket. I was afraid I might not sleep at all if I quit taking my little pills. I devised some strategies to use in place of the prescription medication. Before I stopped taking it, I had a replacement plan in place.

I started taking the over-the-counter supplement melatonin

Do not start any supplement without first discussing it with your physician. Supplements can interfere with certain medications or produce unwanted side effects. Only try melatonin if your doctor indicates that it is a safe option for you. Melatonin has been shown to be effective in restoring the natural sleep cycle in some people suffering from insomnia. According to the information I got about it from my physician, it should never be taken for more than six weeks. That is a sufficient amount of time for resetting natural sleep and wake biorhythms. If you take it for longer than that amount of time, it will do more harm than good because your body will become as dependent on the melatonin as it would be on prescription sleep medication. Taking too much melatonin can cause your body to stop producing natural melatonin which will only make sleep difficulties worse over time.

I stopped taking my prescription sleep medication. Instead I took one 3 mg. tablet of melatonin two hours before I planned to go to bed since it takes about two hours for the melatonin to get into your system. Discuss the appropriate dosage and usage of melatonin with your doctor before taking this supplement.

I created a sleep regimen I could follow every night.
Melatonin, by itself, will not restore natural sleep patterns. I
needed to create a bedtime routine that was simple for me to
follow every night. After dinner, I did not do any work-related
activities. I watched television, checked my Facebook page,
played a fun online game, and relaxed until 11:00 p.m. I took
a warm shower before getting into bed. I grabbed a book and
read until I felt a little sleepy and then turned off the lights.

I wish I could tell you that this worked like magic right away
but the truth is that in the beginning, I often read until 2:00 or
3:00 in the morning before I felt even slightly sleepy. I was not
thrilled about staying awake so late but I was thrilled that I was
eventually actually falling asleep without drugs; so, I continued
my routine. I gradually felt slightly sleepy earlier each night.
After three weeks, I was turning out the lights by 12:00 and
sleeping until 7:00 or 8:00 the next day. Getting seven or eight
hours of natural sleep seemed like a miracle after my three-year
battle with insomnia.

After six weeks, I stopped the melatonin, and continued
the bedtime ritual I had established. I worried the first night
that I didn't take the melatonin that I might not sleep as well
without it. I left it off anyway and waited to see what would
happen. I did my usual routine: started reading at 11:00, turned
out the lights at 12:00, and slept all night. I have been sleeping
soundly ever since. I'm somewhat of a night owl. These days
I am usually in bed by 11:00 or 12:00. I read for an hour or
so until I feel sleepy and usually sleep until 8:00 or 9:00 the
next morning.

I Scheduled Downtime in My Day
As I researched sleep issues, I ran across numerous articles
that said not only do we need to get adequate sleep, but it is
also important for our health to build downtime into our day.
This was an odd concept for me to consider. During the years I

was ill with fibromyalgia, it seemed as if all my days consisted of nothing but downtime.

I felt much better. I had some lingering pain in my legs and knees. Most days, the pain in the rest of my joints and muscles was holding steady at zero. The only variation in the chronic fatigue symptoms was some days I felt like I had the flu and other days I felt like I was recovering from the flu. I felt draggy while I was up and about but I was at long last actually up and about. This coupled with returning to a natural sleep pattern, rather than a pharmaceutically induced one, improved my energy level.

After years of complete inactivity, I was so excited to be able to do things again, that many days I overdid it. I hustled around doing as much as I could while I could because I knew there would be days when I didn't feel like doing anything. I wasn't sure what my present state of health represented. Was I in the early stages of recovery? Was I in remission? Was this a temporary reprieve? I lived in a constant state of fear that not only would my chronic fatigue worsen, but also that all my other fibromyalgia symptoms would come roaring back at any minute.

I was afraid if I stopped to rest, I would never get up again. My pattern was to spend the days that I felt okay running around like a maniac cramming in as much activity as possible. This was inevitably followed by spending several days in bed recovering from the over activity. This was a horrible and unsustainable plan. Eventually, I stepped back and assessed the situation. I needed to schedule intentional downtime into my daily routine. I needed to plan time for rest every single day, no matter how I felt on any given day.

Everyone needs time for rest during the busyness of the day. The form this downtown takes shifts as we pass through different life stages. It is impacted by our age, work hours, parenting responsibilities, current health level, church and community involvement, personal interests, and a hundred other factors in our unique lifestyles.

We find time for everything that is important to us no matter how busy we are. If we want to optimize the potential for recovery from chronic illness and move toward building a healthy lifestyle, we have to create downtime for rest despite our hectic schedules.

When I was in my early twenties, a popular preacher and conference leader, Vance Havner, spoke at my church. I still remember him saying, "We must come apart and rest a while, or we will surely come apart."

That sentiment resonated with me because at the time, Vic and I were newlyweds. We only had one car. Vic was in medical school and I was teaching first grade. Vic was on a demanding surgical rotation. I had to drop him off at med school at 5:00 a.m., come back to our apartment and get ready for my day, drive across town to my school, teach my class, drive back across town, take care of all the household responsibilities, and pick Vic up when he finally finished his day at around 11:00 p.m. It was after midnight by the time we got home and crawled into bed. I was most surely about to come apart.

I took the preacher's advice. (Hello, all you pastors out there. We do listen sometimes.) I restructured the part of my day that was flexible. I had been filling up all the time between when I got home from teaching and when I had to go pick up Vic with activity: grading papers, making lesson plans, running errands, and household chores. I ditched that hectic scenario. I planned a time of rest for an hour each afternoon. Instead of jumping right into household chores as soon as I got home from my teaching job, I made myself a cup of tea and curled up on the couch with a book and did nothing but read, sip, and chill. I came apart and rested for a while and that helped keep me from coming apart during those chaotic days.

I was at a different life stage and a different health stage now. My life had been disrupted by fibromyalgia. I had found ways to improve my symptoms. I didn't want to undo all the progress I had achieved during the past year. I did three things when I stepped back to consider how best to balance work and activity with planned time for rest and relaxation.

Reality Assessment

I realistically assessed my current state of health. Although my fibromyalgia symptoms were vastly improved, I still had pain in some muscles and joints and I still had chronic fatigue that was worse some days than others. But I also had a lot of days where both the pain and fatigue were diminished. On those days, I was doing way too much. I crammed every chore, errand, and household task I could manage into those days. I tossed in church activities and community events. I met friends for lunch. I was doing something from the time I got up until the time I went to bed. I paid for my stubborn insistence on too much activity. Every single time I overdid it on one day, I woke up the next day barely able to move. This wasn't a smart plan for the long haul. Something had to give.

Responsibilities Assessment

I looked at my life and divided my responsibilities into things that had to be done and things that could wait until later. I looked at all the church, community, and social activities I enjoyed. Instead of trying to cram everything into the days I happened to feel a little better, I spread all the things I needed or wanted to do over several weeks. I scheduled when I planned to do each activity on my calendar. I decided to err on the side of doing too little instead of too much. I wrote down wash the towels on Monday, not wash six loads of laundry. I wrote help with ESL (English as a Second Language) classes on Tuesday morning rather than attend every ministry activity at my church that week. And I left a lot of days blank with nothing scheduled at all.

Relaxation Assessment

I needed to plan intentional downtime. But I didn't want to just flop down on the couch or climb into the recliner and stare at the wall. I had done plenty of that at the height of my illness. I thought about relaxing activities that I enjoyed. My one criterion was that whatever I chose could not be related to work, chores, or community activities. It had to be something I did just for fun and just for me.

What are your favorite relaxing activities? Do you have hobbies or pastimes that you particularly enjoy? Do you like gardening, birdwatching, quilting, reading?

I like to play Scrabble. In the past, I participated in competitive Scrabble tournaments all over the country. I even went to the National Scrabble Tournament one year. That wasn't feasible while I was sick. But I could play Scrabble online with actual opponents. I made time to play at least one online game per day. I played on days I felt bad, on days I felt reasonably well, on days I was busy, on days I had nothing scheduled at all. It's amazing how much fun I had and how much I looked forward to Scrabble time.

Doing something you enjoy is not a waste of time. It's a powerful tool for relaxation that refreshes you to do the work you have to do the rest of the day. Now that I'm feeling better, some days I'm tempted to skip my downtime. But I don't. Planning time for rest is important for everyone.

Dr. Norman Drops By

Adequate sleep is an indispensable part of good health. Most healthy adults require seven to nine hours of sleep per night. If you are getting adequate sleep, you wake up feeling refreshed in the morning. Getting too much or too little sleep can make you feel sluggish and tired when you wake up.

Fibromyalgia and chronic fatigue syndrome leave you feeling unrested no matter how much sleep you get. Lack of proper sleep is not only detrimental to good health; it also makes any disease state worse.

As you think about creating a good sleep pattern as part of your chronic illness recovery plan or as a part of establishing a healthy living plan, here are some things to consider.

Insomnia is a component of certain disease states.
Even though it seems illogical that a disease that causes so much fatigue can also cause insomnia, insomnia is a very common component of fibromyalgia,

When you have physical or mental fatigue, normally getting a good night's rest takes away the fatigue and makes you feel refreshed. The brain has a normal sleeping and waking cycle that is often lost in disease states which are characterized by inflammation. This is especially true with fibromyalgia. The sleep disturbances in fibromyalgia include difficulty falling asleep, difficulty staying asleep, waking up in the middle of the night, and waking up unrefreshed.

A vicious cycle of sleep problems can develop in patients with fibromyalgia. The pain which does not allow one to get comfortable leads to decreased sleep. The lack of sleep causes increased fatigue. The increased fatigue causes increased pain which then goes on to cause less sleep. This vicious cycle can only be broken by getting rid of the inflammation. The first step toward ending the cycle of sleep disruption is to get rid of the factors that cause the inflammation. We have given you many concrete suggestions for ways to reduce the inflammation in your body. You need to implement all of these steps before attempting to reset your sleep pattern.

You may need to have a sleep study done.
Although insomnia is a common component of fibromyalgia and other chronic illnesses, sleep disturbances can also be caused by a wide spectrum of pathologies including sleep apnea, thyroid

disease, neurological diseases, and respiratory obstructive diseases. Your doctor may recommend you have a sleep study done by a specialist in this area to determine if you have sleep apnea or other pathologies that are disrupting your normal sleep pattern. A pulmonologist or a physician that specializes in treating sleep disorders will evaluate your specific results. Some disruptive sleep patterns can be treated. For example, sleep apnea often resolves with the nightly use of a CPAP machine. You may need to have a sleep study to evaluate whether, in addition to the insomnia that is often a component of fibromyalgia, you also have a sleep problem that is treatable.

There are health hazards in overscheduling.

A healthy person who tries to cram too much activity into his day is more susceptible to infections and increases his risk for developing elevated blood pressure, indigestion, irritability, difficulty focusing, muddled thinking, lower back pain, neck pain, shoulder pain, and increased anxiety. It is important for everyone to find a balance between activity and rest. This is even more essential for a person dealing with fibromyalgia or another chronic illness.

You may need to decrease your consumption of caffeine.

Caffeine is a stimulant that can easily disrupt sleep patterns, especially if it is consumed later in the day. A general rule of thumb is to consume nothing that contains caffeine after midday. The amount of caffeine consumed in the morning should be monitored. It is recommended to drink no more than one or two cups of coffee or tea per day or the equivalent of other caffeine containing beverages or foods.

Creating a nighttime routine promotes beneficial sleep.

Eliminating harmful chemicals from your home environment and eliminating processed food that is full of chemicals from your diet are important steps for ridding the body of inflammation and optimizing the possibility of recovery from fibromyalgia and other chronic illnesses.

If your sleep pattern has been disrupted by your chronic illness, finding a way to reset your sleep pattern is also important. There are several things you can do to help establish a healthy sleep routine.

- Go to bed at the same time each night.
- Avoid caffeine after midday
- Take a warm bath or shower before getting into bed.
- Do not watch television or look at electronic devices after you get into be. Read a book after you get into bed until you start to feel sleepy.
- Complete a relaxation breathing technique after you turn off the light. This is a simple relaxation breathing technique to do when you are ready to try to go to sleep for the night. Breathe in through your nose while you count to eight. Hold your breath while you count to six. Blow the breath out through your mouth slowly while you count to four. Repeat this breathing exercise if you wake up during the night or if you experience early morning awakening.

Your Turn

1. Evaluate your current sleep pattern. Is insomnia one of your fibromyalgia syndrome symptoms? How many hours of sleep do you get per night? Do you feel rested when you wake up in the morning? List any sleep issues you have, such as, difficulty falling asleep, staying asleep, early morning wakening, wakening in the middle of the night, feeling unrefreshed when you get up.

2. If you have difficulty with sleep, schedule an appointment with your family physician to discuss having a sleep study performed. Write the date of your appointment. Describe the results of any testing done and any treatment options recommended.

3. Create a plan for scheduling downtime into your day. Write down what your plan is for each day for a week. You can do the same thing each day or choose a different relaxing activity each day. Pick something that you enjoy that is just for you. Implement your plan.

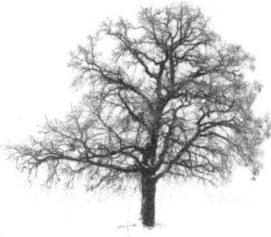

Priority 12: Analyze Your Unique Results

I T TOOK ALMOST a year for me to discover all of the changes I needed to make to create an environment conducive to recovery and then find the most practical ways to incorporate those strategies into my everyday routine. I was on a constant learning curve. After I understood that we live in a toxic world, found my focus, discovered facts about fibromyalgia, dealt with depression, relied on my support group, exchanged harmful household products for safer ones, eliminated most processed foods from my diet, made smart real food choices, added exercise to my day, and reset my sleep cycle; I experienced a remarkable reduction in my fibromyalgia symptoms. Since I was just hoping to find a way to manage my symptoms better, I was amazed by the ultimate outcome of my personal research project.

It took time for my body to detoxify from lifelong exposure to harmful chemicals in household products and processed food. It took time to eat a sufficient amount of real food with anti-oxidants to rev up my immune system and anti-inflammatory nutrients to decrease the inflammation and pain.

People suffering from fibromyalgia have unique symptom patterns and have been ill for varying periods of time. There are different degrees of healing and varying patterns of improvement. Here are few suggestions for evaluating your unique results as you implement the practical priorities for creating a healthier reality.

- Consult your physician before making any lifestyle changes. Keep taking your current medications unless your doctor tells you to discontinue them.
- Take all the time you need to implement each priority. You know yourself, your energy level, and your limitations better than anyone else. Incorporate the recommended changes at a pace that is comfortable for you. You may make one change and then take a break and not make any additional changes for weeks at a time. If that is your particular personal pace, that's fine. The key is to hold steady with the changes you have made. Don't go backwards and don't give up. When you are ready, add the next practical priority and make the next lifestyle change.
- Decide the most practical order for incorporating each change. I shared the changes I made in the chronological order they occurred in my own life. If it is more practical for you to do them in another order, go for it. Do what suits you best. It's your life and your decision.
- Eventually, incorporate every suggested change. To optimize the possibility for recovery, you have to eliminate as many toxic chemicals from your home environment as possible by choosing less toxic household products, cleaning items, cosmetics, and personal care products. You have to stop eating most processed food and add real foods full of antioxidants and anti-inflammatory nutrients to your daily diet. The plan won't work if you ditch processed food but keep using products with fragrance. It won't work if you get rid of toxic cleaning products

but refuse to give up processed food. It won't work if you eliminate as many chemicals as possible but don't eat a lot of real food full of the nutrients you need to decrease inflammation and ramp up your immune system. Do the steps at your own pace in your own way but make a commitment to ultimately do all of them, if it is physically possible for you to do so.

- If you have another chronic illness or physical injury that prevents you from doing every single one of the priorities, make every change that is possible for you. I've met folks that can't eat all the whole foods recommended due to chronic intestinal issues. However, they can eliminate most processed food and eat whatever real foods that their condition allows. I've met other people who have injuries that hinder their ability to do certain types of exercise. However, they have been able to find some sort of movement to add to their day. All of them have improved by making the lifestyle changes that they were able to make.

- After you have completed every step and implemented all of the changes recommended, continue the practical priorities plan for three months. This will give your body the time it needs to completely detoxify and to add the nutrients from real food needed to boost your immune system and reduce inflammation. Usually, ninety days is sufficient time for most people to notice significant improvement.

- At the end of three months, assess how you feel. Do you have fewer symptoms? Are the remaining symptoms less severe? It will be an adventure to see where the journey toward fibromyalgia recovery takes you.

For me, it's been quite a trek. Along the way I struggled not only with my physical health, but also with my faith which had been my anchor and my rock for five decades. I questioned why this had happened to me, wondered about the truth of spiritual life, got mad, and, for a time, completely gave up on myself and on my faith.

It was unrealistic to expect that my life would be completely free of problems. God never promises that to anyone. He just promises to be with us in the mess and chaos. It was equally unrealistic to expect that I could live with reckless disregard for my health without suffering the consequences of my neglect.

I was woefully uninformed about the dangers of our toxic world before I was diagnosed with fibromyalgia. I would have remained that way if I hadn't been desperate to find a way to feel better. The responsibility for creating a chemical-free life was mine to implement or to ignore. I had the freedom to choose and I chose to try.

I embarked on my personal research project. I read everything I could find about fibromyalgia, searched for sources of toxic exposure, and made lifestyle changes hoping to cope with my awful symptoms. This was not a neatly organized linear process. There was a lot of trial and error as I slowly discovered strategies that might help and gradually added specific changes to my daily routine. It was like working a jigsaw puzzle without having the picture on the box top to know what the completed puzzle would look like.

By December of 2012, I had been making lifestyle changes for nearly a year and all of the pieces of the puzzle were finally in place. I just didn't know it yet.

I had made each practical lifestyle change a consistent priority in my daily life. I was encouraged because the fibromyalgia pain was much improved and other symptoms including breathing problems, numbness, dizziness, and fibro fog had completely resolved. I still had chronic fatigue and moderate to severe pain in my legs and knees. I did not have any pain at all in my other muscles and joints.

I was thankful for each positive improvement. Even so, by that December, I felt stymied and stuck. No matter what I tried, the chronic fatigue symptoms and the pain in my knees and legs persisted. This was a limiting factor in my ability to function normally. It was disheartening to think that after almost an entire year of hard work this might be as good as it was going to get.

My spirit had been as bruised and damaged as my body during the years of dealing with chronic illness. Before I got so sick, I routinely read the Bible, prayed, and perused books and articles written by spiritual authors that gave me insight into living a life of faith. During the previous year, I focused most of my time on my research project and expended my daily allotment of energy struggling to cope with my symptoms. Although I was hesitant about plunging headlong back into unwavering faith, I read the occasional scripture passage or a short devotional. For the most part, my Bible spent more time on the shelf than in my hands, my prayers were sporadic and involved a lot of complaining, and I neglected my stack of faith-based reading material.

One of the things I had ignored was sermons written by my daughter's college friend, Dr. Chris George, who is currently pastor of Smoke Rise Baptist Church in Georgia. Chris has a unique and encouraging vision of life and faith. He consistently sent sermons to those on his email list but I was in no mood to read any of them. I mechanically moved each one that arrived from my inbox to my saved files and soon forgot them.

And then this happened. On December 5, 2012, as I lolled in bed contemplating the day ahead, I thought about how much consistently reading encouraging faith words in the morning used to bless my heart and mind. I had made sporadic dives into the morning faith read here and there during the past year. But it had been so long since I ditched the daily habit that I wasn't sure where I wanted to start. Should I read a Bible passage? Find a devotional book? After breakfast, I rifled through my saved email files looking for ideas. I saw all the saved sermons from Chris and randomly clicked one open.

I relate best to sermons that relate to life. No matter how antiquated, odd, convoluted, or irrelevant a scripture passage seems at first glance, I look for practical life application. Chris has a gift for giving Bible passages relevance for today. The sermon I arbitrarily grabbed was entitled, "Hot, Humid, and Hungry." Chris had preached the sermon at First Baptist Church, Mobile, Alabama, where he was pastor at the time, on August 12, 2012. I don't think it was a coincidence that I read that hot and humid sermon on a chilly day in December. It dovetailed with my life experiences during the past year.

The sermon was based on an involved and interesting story found in 1 Kings 19:4-8. This particular scripture passage gives a vivid glimpse into a specific moment in the life of the prophet Elijah. Elijah had just confronted the priests of the Canaanite god Baal in a showdown where he prevailed and they lost. This ticked off their leaders, Queen Jezebel and King Ahab, who swore to capture Elijah and kill him to avenge the honor of the prophets of Baal. Elijah heard they were out to get him. He ran away as far as he could go. When he was exhausted and out of breath, he hunkered down beneath a broom tree in the desert.

Chris writes: "Elijah did what anyone would do confronted with this situation. He ran...He felt isolated and ostracized, persecuted and threatened. He may have struggled with doubt, depression...Sitting under the broom tree, he must have wondered, 'Why am I here? What can I do?'"

I was intrigued. I wasn't sitting under a broom tree. I was sitting on my couch. I had seen God do wonderful things in my life in the past just like Elijah had. But in this present moment I felt isolated, threatened, and depressed by the lingering symptoms of fibromyalgia. And I wondered, "Why am I here?" Here at this place still dealing with chronic illness and the inability to function normally. I thought, "What can I do?" I had acted on every piece of information I found to make changes to create a chemical-free life and move toward a healthier outcome. After all that effort, I wondered what I was going to do with the rest of my life. My ability to function normally was still compromised by fibromyalgia.

I stopped reading and tried to pray. I asked God to show me how I could find meaning for the rest of my life if the remaining pain and the chronic fatigue symptoms never went away. I felt sorry for myself just like Elijah. I longed for a broom tree so that I would have a suitable spot to sit and be miserable and pout.

In an attempt to shake off my negative mood, I made a gratitude list of the positive things that had happened during the past year. I still had moderate to severe pain in my knees and legs but no pain in my other muscles and joints. I was able to leave the house and do a few things now. I was exhausted when I got home and it took days to recuperate but at least I was able to do more. I still was alive and in the world. If chronic illness was going to be my constant companion for the rest of my life, I wanted to find a way to accept that as my new normal. I longed to remember how to exercise my faith muscles which had atrophied from lack of use as surely as my physical muscles had. I asked God to show me how to trust him to get me through one day at a time. I felt a sense of peace wash over me after this pause for prayer and reflection.

I was in the middle of the sermon but I had a lot to think about already. So, I laid the sermon down and got up and got on with my day. I contemplated Elijah and broom trees, despair and gratitude, effort and outcomes, as I puttered around the house completing my chores for the day.

That night before climbing into bed, I plopped down on the couch to read the rest of Chris's sermon. In the next paragraph he said, "We may not have the same experiences as...Elijah, but all of us at some moment have struggled with this same despair and asked these same questions. We too have grown weary trying to do the right things, only to experience more obstacles and feel threatened by the world around us." Well, I could certainly say amen to that. I had tried to do the right things to get healthier but I still felt threatened by the limitations my illness caused in my life.

I kept reading. Elijah ran away from what threatened him and ended up in the wilderness. He found a smidgen of shade under a scraggly broom tree and sat down beneath it to mope. Chris continued with his thoughts, "The wilderness is a dangerous place that supports little life. The wilderness is never anyone's destination. We travel through the wilderness in our lives only when absolutely necessary, when we have no other choice."

Exactly! I certainly didn't want the wilderness of compromised health to be the only destination I had left for the rest of my life. Elijah was hot and tired and afraid in his wilderness to the point that he asked God just to let him die. God listened to Elijah's complaints just like he had been listening to me for months, just like he listens to all of us wherever we are, whatever our circumstances. We may be sick or well, ready to make changes to get healthy. or reluctant to change anything at all. God listens. God cares.

I was mesmerized by now as I continued reading. I read through several more paragraphs until I got to the part where God speaks to Elijah through a messenger, in some translations referred to as an angel, that he sends to bring him food and water. When I read the words that the messenger spoke to Elijah, I was stunned because every single word was like a promise from God directly to me.

Chris said the messenger had specific instructions from God for Elijah. He told him: "Get up. Your journey is not over. Get up. I have a plan for your life. Get up. I have somewhere for you to go, something for you to do. Get up. Eat. Get ready."

By the time I read those words for the third time, tears were rolling down my cheeks. It sounds weird, even to me, as I write this down; but somehow those long-ago words from that ancient story triggered the conviction that my remaining symptoms would resolve. It might be months or years away, but I knew down to the very core of my being that better days were ahead somewhere down the road. I had places to go and things to do and was sure I would get there one day out in the future.

It was late. The only place left to go that night was to bed. So, I did. The next morning, on December 6, 2012, a shaft of brilliant sunlight pierced through the blinds and woke me from a deep sleep. I threw the covers back, sat up, swung my legs over the edge of the bed, and stood up.

I was still half asleep as I stumbled to the bathroom to wash my face and brush my teeth. I turned on the lights. And then I stopped and stood very still with my hand frozen on the light switch. I was suddenly fully awake because I had just realized something quite strange. For the first time in three years there was absolutely no pain in any of my joints or muscles. There was no pain at all, even in my knees and legs, which had never stopped hurting – until now. And the debilitating flu-like chronic fatigue was gone. I felt completely normal.

I had been confident the night before that the remainder of my symptoms would eventually resolve. It had not occurred to me that I would wake up symptom free the very next morning.

I couldn't process this. I was so used to feeling horrible all of the time that I scarcely knew what to do with myself feeling well. I woke up every morning for weeks afterward wondering if this was some kind of temporary reprieve, wondering if this might be the day that the symptoms returned. But they haven't.

Today, all these years later, here I sit at the keyboard still completely symptom free. I continue to read and research additional ways to get chemicals out of my home and food. I do what I can to avoid exposure to toxic substances in things I use every day. I still avoid most processed food and continue to find out everything I can about which whole foods are the most nutritious and helpful in keeping my body healthy.

I find new articles every week about doctors and scientists doing research on the link between chemical exposure in our homes and processed foods and all kinds of chronic illness. I hear about other people who have recovered from a variety of illnesses from doing the same things I did.

So, I wanted to share my story with you. If you have fibromyalgia, I want to encourage you that there is hope. You can get better. Your symptoms can improve. You may even completely recover. I did.

If you aren't currently ill, the strategies shared in this book can help you prevent the onset of chronic illness and create a healthier life for yourself and your family.

It is my sincerest wish that this book will be helpful to every single person who wants to create a chemical-free life to optimize health in our toxic world. I want to remind you that you are strong and capable and can do anything you put your mind to do. It is my prayer that the lifestyle changes you make will truly change your life.

When I started my personal research project, I hoped I would find something to improve my symptoms. I had no expectation that I would completely recover. Even as my pain improved in gradual increments, I thought there would always be some lingering effects. I never internalized the possibility that every symptom might eventually resolve until the day I sat down to read these words from Chris's sermon:

"Get up. Your journey is not over. Get up. I have a plan for your life. Get up. I have somewhere for you to go, something for you to do. Get up. Eat. Get ready."

How about you? You may not be into sermons and your faith touchstones might be different than mine. Whatever else you happen to believe, please have confidence in your power to change the trajectory of your illness. If you choose to implement the practical priorities for recovery shared in this book, hold tight to whatever gives you motivation and strength. Prepare for a whirlwind trek that may take you to unexpected destinations. I don't know where your personal journey will lead. But I know this. There is somewhere for you to go. There is something for you to do. Get up. Get ready.

Dr. Norman Drops By

When I graduated from medical school and completed my residency in family practice in the seventies, there was not a name for fibromyalgia. I don't recall seeing a single case of what now would be described as a patient with a fibromyalgia syndrome pattern during those years. By the time I returned to the United States from working in a mission hospital in Colombia and went into private practice in the late eighties, I began to see patients with a fibromyalgia type pattern. Sometimes this was called fibrositis or chronic fatigue syndrome but the symptom pattern was typical for fibromyalgia.

In the mid to late nineties, I began to see a significant increase in the number of patients who came to my office with fibromyalgia type symptoms. There was no consensus for a recommended treatment plan at that time. Various treatments were used including medications to control the pain, antidepressants, and medications that sedated the nerve pain pathways to the brain.

When I retired from private practice and began teaching medical students in 2011, new scientific investigations into fibromyalgia showed that it is an inflammatory process disease centered on abnormal responses in the nerve pathways. Researchers suspected that this inflammation was exacerbated by exposure to toxins in the environment and in the chemicals in processed food. The students I worked with attended lectures describing the connections between eating too much processed food full of potentially toxic chemicals and all kinds of disease processes, including fibromyalgia. This period of time overlapped the same period of time that Kathy started her personal research project to find a way to improve her symptoms after being diagnosed with fibromyalgia.

There is still no definitive picture of the cause and cure for fibromyalgia. What we do know now is that inflammation plays a significant role in fibromyalgia symptoms, that exposure to chemicals increases inflammation in the body, and that reducing exposure to toxic chemicals reduces inflammation.

If I was still in practice, I would recommend that all my patients with fibromyalgia do what Kathy did. I would devise a treatment plan that centers on decreasing chemical exposure. I saw with my own eyes how much Kathy improved by implementing each of the practical priorities for fibromyalgia recovery. There is a significant improvement in symptoms for fibromyalgia patients who eliminate household products made with toxic chemicals from their home environment, stop eating processed food, and eat a diet that emphasizes foods with antioxidants and anti-inflammatory nutrients. Today Kathy remains free of fibromyalgia symptoms.

Looking back and analyzing what occurred, I feel that the cause of Kathy's fibromyalgia onset was a combination of factors including genetic predisposition, the trigger event of a severe allergic reaction, and lifelong exposure to toxic chemicals. Eliminating chemicals helped detoxify her body. Eating real food full of antioxidants boosted her immune system. Eating food with anti-inflammatory nutrients helped decrease the inflammation caused by the disease process.

Most fibromyalgia patients should see significant improvement following this plan. It is possible to completely recover. The research is ongoing and there is new scientific evidence every day that confirms this.

I walked alongside Kathy every step of the way during her journey with fibromyalgia. As a physician, I can confidently recommend implementing the practical priorities as a viable treatment plan for improving fibromyalgia symptoms.

Your Turn

1. Look at the recipes for nontoxic cleaners in Appendix I. Choose one cleaner to make this week. Write down the product you exchange, which safer version you choose, and the date you made the switch. Repeat this process for other items in the appendix that interest you.

2. Look at the recipes and suggestions for making real food convenient in Appendix II. Use the recipes and suggestions to plan menus for the coming week. Write down which recipe you use and the date. Repeat the process for other recipes in the appendix that interest you.

3. After you have implemented all of the priorities for fibromyalgia recovery and have done them all consistently for three months, look back to the symptom list you created at the end of the first chapter. Cross off any symptoms that have completely resolved. For any remaining symptoms, rate how much that particular symptom has improved on a scale of one to ten, with one being minimum improvement and ten being maximum improvement. This will give you a clear picture of your personal progress toward recovery. Describe any improvements you have noticed.

Appendix I Recipes for Nontoxic Cleaners and Household Products

You can buy nontoxic household products from companies that are dedicated to using safer ingredients like Method and Seventh Generation. You can find organic substitutes for products you routinely use. One of my favorite finds is organic wool dryer balls. They are a unique natural replacement for industrially manufactured fabric softeners and dryer sheets that often contain harmful chemical ingredients. The dryer balls not only soften your laundry, they also reduce the drying time for each load. Another great option is to make cleaners, pest removers, and other household products yourself using inexpensive ingredients you probably already have on hand or can easily purchase.

This is a starter list for ingredients that can be used to make multiple products.

- Baking soda. Buy the big boxes in the cleaning section instead of the small boxes in the baking section to get the most bang for your buck.
- Borax. You can find it in the laundry supplies section of the store.
- Castile soap. It is made from olive oil. It is organic, nontoxic, biodegradable, and will not harm the environment. It can be purchased from Amazon.com or other online retailers, your favorite big box store, health food stores, camping stores, and hiking stores. I use Castile for any

recipe that calls for liquid soap. If you prefer, substitute your favorite nontoxic dishwashing liquid.
- Hydrogen peroxide. Save money by buying big bottles of the least expensive brand at discount stores.
- Vinegar. Buy plain white vinegar in large size jugs at discount or big box stores.

Here are some recipes for some of my favorite home-made nontoxic cleaners, pest repellents, and other household products.

Cleaning Products

All-Purpose Cleaner
Fill a spray bottle with half plain white vinegar and half water. Spray the solution onto the surface you want to clean. Wipe off the solution with a paper towel or a microfiber cloth.

Vinegar at this concentration kills as many germs as most commercial products. I use this mixture to clean surfaces in the bathroom and kitchen, counter tops, mirrors, chrome fixtures, doorknobs, light switches, appliances, the stove top, sinks, and anywhere else you would use an all-purpose cleaner. I use a microfiber cloth, rather than paper towels, when cleaning mirrors, windows, and other glass surfaces to prevent streaking.

Drain Cleaner
Pour 1/4 cup of baking soda down the drain. Add 1 cup of vinegar. It will bubble and foam when you add the vinegar. Let the mixture sit for one hour. Run cold water down the drain for a few minutes to flush.

If you have a drain in your sink or shower that gets stopped up, you can use vinegar and baking soda to remove the clog. Use ½ cup of baking soda and two cups of vinegar for stopped up drains. Let the mixture sit overnight and flush with cold water in the morning.

Floor Cleaner for Tile

Mix the following ingredients in a one-gallon plastic pitcher with a pouring spout:

2 teaspoons of liquid Castile soap

½ cup of baking soda

1 gallon of warm water

½ cup of white vinegar

Put the liquid dish soap, baking soda, and half the warm water into the pitcher and mix well with a large spoon. Then add the vinegar. The mixture will bubble up and foam when you add the vinegar. Wait for the foam to subside before adding the rest of the water.

Pour the mixture into a mop that has a reservoir for adding your own cleaning mixture and a removable mop head that you can wash after each use.

I use this floor cleaning mixture on the quarry tile floors in my kitchen, sunroom, den, and foyer and the ceramic tile floors in my bathrooms. Vacuum up loose dirt from the tile and then mop with the cleaning mixture. For the final step, use a clean mop to rinse with clear water.

I am amazed at the amount of dirt that the homemade cleaner removes. The rinse step removes even more dirt. It works better than any commercial cleaning product I have ever used and it's nontoxic.

Another option for cleaning floors without chemicals is a steam floor cleaner that uses only water. There are several types of these machines designed to use for different floor coverings including tile, wood, and carpet. Check to make sure it is okay to use a steamer on your specific type of flooring without causing any damage.

Shower and Bathtub Cleaner

Put 1 cup of Castile liquid soap in a large spray bottle.

Heat 1 cup of plain white vinegar in the microwave until warm. Add to the bottle with the soap and shake to mix.

Spray on shower and tub surfaces. Leave for 1 hour. Scrub and then rinse.

Toilet Bowl Cleaner
Use a funnel to put ingredients in this order into a 16 ounce or larger squirt bottle:
>3 tablespoons of baking soda
>1/3 cup liquid Castile soap
>2 cups of water

Shake the bottle to mix the ingredients thoroughly. Squirt underneath the rim and on the inside surfaces of the toilet bowl. Scrub with a toilet bowl brush and rinse.

Whirlpool Tub Jet Cleaner
Have you ever settled into your whirlpool tub anticipating a relaxing bath only to be slimed by gunk shooting out from the jets when you hit the on switch? Use the following mixture once a month to clean the jets and you will never be slimed again.

Fill the tub with warm water until all of the jets are covered with water. Add 2 cups of borax, 1 cup of baking soda, and 2 quarts of vinegar to the water. Turn on the jets and let them run for 30 minutes. Turn off the jets and leave the water in the tub for several hours or overnight.

Drain the tub and use paper towels to wipe up all of the gunk that has come out of the jets. Fill the tub with cold water and run the jets for 30 minutes. Drain the tub and wipe up any remaining residue.

Spray vinegar and water all-purpose cleaner around the tub and wipe with paper towels or a microfiber cloth to leave the tub clean and sparkling.

Wood Restorer and Cleaner
Mix ¾ cup canola oil and ¼ cup white vinegar with a wire whisk until completely blended. Rub this mixture on any type

of wooden furniture in need of restoration and/or cleaning. Leave it on the piece of furniture overnight. In the morning rub with a clean dry cloth to remove any excess liquid. Depending on the amount of damage, there may not be much liquid left. Pieces that are severely scratched, old, or dry will soak up most of the mixture. Use a dry cloth to buff the furniture to a nice clean shine.

To test how this will work on a specific piece of furniture, rub a little of the mixture into an inconspicuous place on the underside of the furniture, leave overnight, and rub with a clean cloth in the morning. If you are pleased with the test patch, you are ready to do the whole piece. If the furniture has a lot of scratches and marred spots, you may have to repeat the steps.

I have used this on all types of wooden furniture. Here are two examples. I purchased a dining room table at a huge discount because it had been used as a floor model and was covered with scratches and dings. It is made of dark mango wood and rubber wood. I used this mixture

on it twice and all of the scratches disappeared. I reapply the mixture every few months for maintenance and in between times simply dust it and wipe up spills with a damp cloth. I've also used this mixture with great success on two rocking chairs made of a light colored tropical wood that I bought in Colombia thirty-five years ago. The chairs were marred and scratched from years of use and several trips in a moving van. They look like new.

Pest Repellents

Ant Repellent
There are all kinds of natural substances you can use to discourage ants from coming into your house. Use one of the following around windowsills, underneath the sink, by a doorsill, or wherever you notice ants entering your house: lemon juice, vinegar, or cinnamon.

To get rid of ants that are already in your house add 1 or 2 teaspoons of Castile liquid soap to a spray bottle filled with half vinegar and half water. Spray the mixture on any ants you see.

If ants keep coming in, mix 1 tablespoon of borax with 3 tablespoons of confectioner sugar. Put in small containers. Bottlecaps or small jar lids work nicely. Place the containers in the locations where you see ants coming into the house. They will eat this mixture plus take it back to their nest. The ants should be gone within two days.

Mosquito Repellents
There are several ways to control mosquitos without using strong toxic chemicals. Purchase an electronic bug zapper and hang it near an outside seating area. Plant citronella, marigolds, and garlic in pots and place them around your patio. Mix a few drops of oil of peppermint in a spray bottle of warm water. Spritz a small amount of this mixture on your arms and legs.

Moth Repellent
Put cloves and/or bay leaves in a mesh bag. Hang the bag in closets where you want to repel moths. Refill the bags after a few months when the smell of the cloves and/or bay leaves starts to diminish.

Mouse Repellent
Soak cotton balls in pure peppermint oil. Place them wherever you notice mice coming in. The smell discourages them from entering the space.

Other Household Products

Air Freshener
Put baking soda or white vinegar into a small dish. If the odor is particularly strong, use one dish of each. Place in the area

where you want to absorb odors. Leave overnight. Remove the dish the next morning and pour the contents down the sink.

If the odor persists, empty out the dish or dishes and refill it with more vinegar and/or baking soda. Leave in place for an additional night. Repeat as many days as necessary until the odor is gone.

Air Purifier

Houseplants function as natural air purifiers. As part of their growth cycle, they absorb not only carbon dioxide, but also other harmful chemicals including VOCs. Before bringing any plant into your home, make sure it is not poisonous for animals or small children if you have pets or babies. Also check for plants that cause allergies if you have family members who suffer from pollen allergies. Check for cross reactivity to latex if anyone in your home suffers from latex allergies.

The following plants are particularly efficient at purifying air, are easy to find at most plant nurseries, and add decorative touches to your inside spaces: aloe vera, bamboo palm, Boston fern, English ivy, Gerber daisy, mother-in-law's tongue, orchid, peace lily, philodendron, spider plant. When you water the plants, also spritz the leaves with a mister to keep dust from collecting on the leaves.

Garbage Disposal Freshener

Chop up any citrus fruit: lemons, oranges, or limes. Put the fruit in the garbage disposal. Turn the disposal on just long enough to start grinding the fruit.

Leave the partially ground fruit in the disposal for one to two hours. Grind up the fruit completely. Flush with cold water for several minutes.

Kitchen Air Freshener

Put the following ingredients into a small pot and simmer on low on the stovetop to give your kitchen a pleasant chemical free scent.

2 cups of water
1 orange cut into wedges
1 lemon or lime cut into wedges
2 cinnamon sticks

Wallpaper Paste

I had several places in my home where wallpaper was starting to come loose from the wall. We took down some of the wallpaper and painted the walls with VOC free paint. In my guest bedroom the wallpaper still looked nice and matched my decorating scheme. However, the paper was starting to come loose in one corner of the room. We had tried to repair this with a commercial product but it didn't work. After I started getting rid of chemicals in the house, we didn't want to try another commercial product so I made my own wallpaper paste. It worked beautifully! No more loose wallpaper.

In a small bowl mix:

½ cup of flour
2 tablespoons of sugar
Add 1 cup of water slowly.
Beat well with a wire whisk until it is smooth.

Pour the mixture into a small saucepan over medium heat and stir constantly until the mixture comes to a boil. Keep over the heat and continue stirring until the mixture is thick and stiff. Remove from the heat and add 1 teaspoon of alum.

I used a small paintbrush to spread the paste on the underside of the wallpaper that had come loose and onto the part of the wall where I needed to stick it. I used a clean soft cloth to press the seam down and remove any excess paste that came out. You could probably make this in large quantities to paper a whole room from scratch but I only have experience using it to repair loose wallpaper.

Weed Killer

I found this on Pinterest – which is a great resource for nontoxic product ideas. Mix one gallon of vinegar, 2 cups of Epsom salts, and ¼ cup of liquid dish soap in an electric powered sprayer. Mix well. Thoroughly saturate the weeds. Wait a few days to see if the weeds are starting to die off. If needed, spray the area again. This works best when there are just a few weeds coming up. You may have to use something else if you are trying to eradicate weeds from an extremely overgrown area.

If you would like other ideas for making your own household products, the internet is a wonderful resource. Put keywords in your favorite search engine that include the type of cleaner you are looking for plus words like nontoxic, chemical free, or organic. Check out boards on Pinterest. Follow sites on Facebook and Twitter that promote an organic and chemical free lifestyle. Here's to nontoxic chemical-free living for all!

Appendix II Real Food Recipes

Processed food is full of toxic chemicals that make us sick. The only thing it has going for it is speed and convenience. Making food from scratch takes time. Since the thing real food has going for it is health and well-being, I was determined to give it a try. I wanted to get well and stay well. Making real food recipes has certainly been worth the extra time and effort. Besides, over the years I've found a lot of ways to make cooking with real food more convenient.

Ten Tips for Making Real Food Convenient
- Stock your pantry with real food staples.
- Basic starter list: canned beans that have only one ingredient: the beans, organic canned tomatoes and tomato sauce, chicken broth and beef broth with no added chemicals, olive oil, whole wheat flour and unbleached all-purpose flour, baking powder, baking soda, organic raw sugar, ground flaxseed, purple onions, fresh garlic, sweet potatoes.
- Fill your freezer with frozen fruit and veggies.
- Choose brands that have only one ingredient: the fruit or the vegetable.
- Create an anti-inflammatory spice kit.
- Basic starter list: basil, cayenne pepper, chili powder, cilantro, cinnamon, cumin, garlic (fresh), ginger (fresh),

ginger (ground), oregano, pepper to grind, rosemary, sea salt, turmeric
- Plan menus weekly.
- Buy all the ingredients for your weekly plan before you start cooking for the week.
- Keep fresh fruit, raw vegetables, and raw nuts on hand for snacks. Fruit tip: freeze fresh pineapple and grapes for cool crunchy snacks and to use in smoothies. Veggie tip: Slice carrots and celery into small sticks and put them in a container that has a lid. Completely cover the sticks with cold water, snap on the lid and pop them into the refrigerator. They'll last for at least a week.
- Make double batches of everything and freeze the extras in both single and family size serving portions.
- Bake and freeze enough bread to last one to two weeks.
- Cook meat for sandwiches and freeze in single serving portions.
- Grill chicken fingers and hamburger patties in large batches and freeze for a fast food fix.

I'm a fly by the seat of my pants kind of cook. I make a lot of real food dishes without recipes. I concluded my readers might appreciate instructions a tad more specific than toss some things into a bowl until it looks right. Over the past few months, my kitchen has been a test lab as I sorted and measured and considered what I put into each dish. After you get used to cooking from scratch, I hope you will embrace the freedom of recipe free cooking. Don't be afraid to substitute ingredients and experiment with different flavor combinations. I'll give you a few suggestions on how to do that in the recipes I share.

BREAD

You can make any bread recipe healthier by making a few substitutions and additions to the original recipe. Use whole wheat flour instead of white flour for at least half of the flour called for in the recipe. Substitute steel cut oats for part of the flour or toss in a handful of oats in addition to the flour. For sweetener use raw honey, molasses, real maple syrup, or raw organic sugar instead of refined white sugar. Try almond milk or cashew milk instead of whole regular milk. Replace part of the butter called for with coconut oil and/or olive oil. Add ground flaxseed and/or ground chia seed to the dry ingredients. Add nuts, whole seeds, dried fruit, and berries to the recipe.

If you have intolerance to gluten, experiment with gluten free flours such as almond flour, rice flour, tapioca flour, or a mixture of gluten free flours and gluten free steel cut oats. If you do not have gluten intolerance, use the best quality whole grain flour you can find.

If you are lactose intolerant or have a true allergy to dairy products, substitute almond, rice, or soy milk for cow's milk. Replace butter with coconut oil, olive oil, or an organic butter substitute.

If you want to make homemade bread, muffins are a great place to start. They are simple to make. You can turn one basic recipe into lots of flavorful varieties. They are delicious for breakfast, as well as for a quick snack.

Basic Muffin Recipe

Grease a 12-cup muffin tin and preheat the oven to 400 degrees.

Stir together in a medium sized bowl:

1 cup whole wheat flour

3/4 cup unbleached all-purpose flour

1/3 cup raw organic sugar

2 tablespoons ground flaxseed

2 teaspoon baking powder

1/4 teaspoon salt

In a separate small bowl beat together:

2 free range organic eggs

1 tablespoon melted butter

1 tablespoon melted coconut oil

1 teaspoon pure vanilla extract

3/4 cup milk

Make a well in the center of the dry ingredients. Pour the liquid ingredients into the well. Mix together by hand until all ingredients are moist. Don't overmix. It's okay if the batter has a few lumps in it.

Fill the muffin tin with an equal amount of batter for each muffin. Just eyeball this until it looks even to you.

Pop the pan in the oven and bake for 20 to 25 minutes. The muffins are done when the tops are a nice golden brown. If you aren't sure they're done, stick a toothpick in the thickest part of the muffin and pull it out. If the toothpick has nothing sticking to it, the muffins are ready to take out of the oven. Leave them in the pan for three minutes. Run a knife around the edge of each muffin and lift it out of the pan. Place the muffins on a rack to cool completely. Put them in a freezer-safe container or bag and freeze. Take out one at a time as needed. Defrost in the microwave for 45 to 60 seconds and you have a fresh, warm muffin ready to eat.

You can take this basic recipe and turn it into all kinds of yummy muffins. Use your imagination and personal favorite flavor combinations to make any kind of muffin you want. Add fruit, chopped nuts, spices or whatever you like. Here are a few ideas.

Apple Oatmeal Muffins

Use the Basic Muffin Recipe with the following changes and additions.

To the dry ingredients in the Basic Muffin Recipe, add:

½ cup steel cut oats

½ teaspoon ground cinnamon

½ teaspoon ground ginger

½ cup raisins

½ cup chopped walnuts or almonds

1 apple, any variety, peeled and grated

Follow the rest of the directions for the Basic Muffin Recipe.

Banana Nut Tropical Muffins

Use the Basic Muffin Recipe with the following changes and additions.

To the dry ingredients in the Basic Muffin Recipe, add:

¼ cup chopped almonds

¼ cup chopped walnuts

¼ cup grated organic packaged coconut or grated fresh coconut. If you use packaged coconut, look for an organic brand that contains only one ingredient: shredded coconut. Many brands of commercially packaged coconut contain artificial dye added to make it whiter and may contain other unhealthy additives.

Mash one small ripe banana and put it into the well you make in the center of the dry ingredients.

Follow the rest of the directions for the Basic Muffin Recipe.

Blueberry Muffins

Use the Basic Muffin Recipe with the following changes and additions.

Put one cup of fresh or frozen blueberries into a shallow bowl. Sprinkle the berries with 2 T of raw organic sugar and let sit for five minutes.

Follow the directions for the Basic Muffin Recipe. Put the sugared blueberries and any juice that's oozed deliciously out of them into the well you make in the center of the dry ingredients.

Follow the rest of the directions for the Basic Muffin Recipe.

Strawberry Muffins

Use the Basic Muffin Recipe with the following changes and additions.

Hull and slice one cup of fresh or frozen strawberries into a shallow bowl. Sprinkle the berries with 2 tablespoons of raw organic sugar and let sit for five minutes.

Follow the rest of the directions for the Basic Muffin Recipe. Put the sugared berries and any juice that's oozed deliciously out of them into the well you make in the center of the dry ingredients.

Use a wire whisk to add 1 container of strawberry fruit on the bottom organic Greek yogurt to the liquid ingredients.

Follow the rest of the directions for the Basic Muffin Recipe.

If muffins aren't your cup of tea, how about scones? I don't know if I've watched too much "Downton Abbey" and "The Crown "or what. All I know is I love scones, that delightful triangle of deliciousness that is the British version of a southern biscuit. I had bought them at bakeries and eaten them in tearooms but I had no idea I could bake them myself. They are simple to make, lend themselves to a variety of flavors, and I say, old chap, they are quite fun to make and rather tasty!

Basic Scone Recipe

Preheat the oven to 400 degrees and line a large cookie sheet with parchment paper.

In a medium sized bowl, mix:

1 cup whole wheat flour

1 ½ cups unbleached all-purpose flour

¼ cup raw organic sugar

2 tablespoons ground flaxseed

1 tablespoon baking powder

½ teaspoon salt

Cut into the dry ingredients with a pastry cutter:

4 tablespoons chilled butter

2 tablespoons chilled coconut oil

If you don't have a pastry cutter, put it on your shopping list. In the meantime, you can use two knives for this step. Just keep cutting the butter and coconut oil into the dry ingredients until they are in tiny uniform pieces about the size of small peas. Helpful hint: Put the butter and coconut oil in a small bowl in the freezer before you get out the rest of the ingredients and start the recipe and it will be nice and chilled by the time you get to this step.

In a small bowl whisk together:

2 organic free-range eggs

1/3 cup of milk

Make a well in the center of the dry ingredients. Pour the milk and egg mixture into the well and stir with a spoon. Then, use your hands to finish mixing. Keep squishing the ingredients together with your hands until they are completely mixed and you have a nice soft ball of dough.

Divide the dough into two balls of equal size.

Sprinkle flour on a large cutting board or two large round plates. Pretend you are a famous British pastry chef as you flatten each ball of dough into a round disc on the floured cutting board. Hum British tunes as you flip the discs over so both sides have flour on them. Think about your favorite British royal as you shape the balls into two beautiful flat circles about a ½ inch thick.

Pour ¼ cup milk into a bowl or cup. Dip a pastry brush into the milk and brush the top of each disc with milk. Sprinkle 1 tablespoon of raw organic sugar evenly over the milk on top of each disc. The milk will absorb the sugar.

Cut each disc into eight triangles. Put the triangles on the parchment paper lined cookie sheet. Bake for 20 minutes or until golden brown on the bottom and just starting to brown on the tops.

Remove from oven and leave on the cookie sheet for two minutes. Take them off the cookie sheet and cool completely on a wire rack.

You can freeze them the same way as the muffins and remove from the freezer and defrost as needed. Serve the scones warm as is or with butter, raw local honey, or your favorite jelly. If you are feeling really British, serve them with clotted cream and your favorite jam.

Like muffins, scones lend themselves to lots of yummy variations. Here are a few ideas.

Blueberry Scones

Use the Basic Scones Recipe with the following changes and additions.

Put one cup of fresh or frozen blueberries into a shallow bowl. Sprinkle the berries with 2 T of raw organic sugar and let sit for five minutes.

Stir the berries into the dry ingredients after you cut in the butter and before making the well in the center to add the liquid ingredients.

Add 1 teaspoon of pure vanilla extract to the liquid ingredients.

Follow the rest of the directions in the Basic Scones Recipe.

Cinnamon Scones

Use the Basic Scones Recipe with the following changes and additions.

Use ¼ cup of organic dark brown sugar instead of ¼ cup raw organic sugar.

Add 2 teaspoons of ground cinnamon to the dry ingredients.

Add ½ teaspoon cinnamon to 2 tablespoons of raw organic sugar. Mix well. Sprinkle half of this mixture on the top of each disc after you have brushed on the milk.

Follow the rest of the directions for the Basic Scone Recipe.

Lemon Poppyseed Scones

Use the Basic Scones Recipe with the following changes and additions.

Add to the dry ingredients:

1 tablespoon of poppyseeds

The zest from two lemons. The zest is the colorful part of the fruit rind. Scrape off just the colored part and not the white layer underneath the rind as the white part can be quite bitter. If you don't have a citrus zester, add it to your shopping list. It's a handy kitchen tool for adding zest from any citrus fruit to a recipe. In the meantime, you can use the tip of a small sharp knife to carefully scrape off the zest.

Use lemon juice for the liquid instead of milk. Put a small strainer on top of a measuring cup and squeeze the juice from both lemons into the cup. If you do not have enough lemon juice to equal 1/3 cup, add additional freshly squeezed lemon juice or bottled lemon juice to the measuring cup until you have 1/3 cup of total liquid.

Follow the rest of the directions in the Basic Scone Recipe.

Orange Cranberry Scones

Use the Basic Scones Recipe with the following changes and additions.

Add to the dry ingredients:

½ cup of dried cranberries

The zest from one large orange. The zest is the colorful part of the fruit rind. Scrape off just the colored part and not the white layer underneath the rind as the white part can be quite bitter. If you don't have a citrus zester, add it to your shopping list. It's a handy kitchen tool for adding zest from any citrus fruit to a recipe. In the meantime, you can use the tip of a small sharp knife to carefully scrape off the zest.

Use orange juice for the liquid instead of milk. Put a small strainer on top of a measuring cup and squeeze the juice from the orange you just zested into the cup. If you do not have enough orange juice to equal 1/3 cup, add bottled orange juice to the measuring cup until you have 1/3 cup of total liquid. Use a brand that is 100% orange juice with no added chemicals.

After you shape the discs, brush the top of each disc with orange juice instead of milk.

Follow the rest of the directions in the Basic Scone Recipe

There are many other kinds of bread you can make. I make gingerbread, banana bread, whole wheat loaf bread, cinnamon raisin bread, and more. Look for bread recipes online and in your favorite cookbooks. Make any recipe you find healthier by making the substitutions and additions described at the beginning of the bread section.

You may want to buy some bread. The first year I switched from processed food to eating real food, I was determined to make all the bread I ate. I made loaf bread to slice, sandwich buns, bagels, and every single type of bread I put into my mouth.

I wanted all my priorities to be practical and I couldn't keep up that pace. I got 12 to 14 slices out of a loaf of sandwich bread.

I could make that last a week or so for just the two of us. It was gone in a day if the grandkids dropped by for lunch. The sandwich buns were yummy but one batch yielded only eight to ten buns and they were labor intensive even when I used a bread machine for kneading. Homemade bagels are delicious but making them requires multiple steps that took up most of a day to make.

I didn't have the time nor the energy to make all my bread plus cook everything else from scratch too. Honestly, I don't know how those pioneer women did it in their little log cabins in the woods.

Remember my 90%-10% goal for eating real food? Some bread makes up a part of the 10% of processed food I eat each day. I look for brands that contain the most natural real ingredients and the fewest chemical additives. One of my favorite brands is Ezekiel Bread. It is made from organic ingredients and has no artificial additives. It's not available in my small rural town. So, sometimes I just go to my local supermarket, read the ingredient labels, and buy the brand that is the healthiest choice from the options available.

Another product that falls into the bread category is cereal. Boxed cereal is another processed food that people use frequently due to its convenience. If you want to continue using prepackaged cereal, be sure to look for brands that have the fewest ingredients and the fewest added chemicals. There are several companies that make organic cereals and granola. Several options to check out are Kashi, Ezekiel, Cascadian Farms, and Nature's Path. These brands are like everything you buy in a box. You have to read the ingredients labels and see what is in the cereal. Anyone can slap the words organic and natural on the box and the product still may contain unwanted chemicals.

Granola is something that is easy to make yourself. Once you have the basic recipe down, it is simple to make different flavor combinations by adding different combinations of dry and liquid ingredients plus a variety of dried fruits, chopped nuts, and spices.

Granola

The formula for making any type of granola involves four simple steps.

Mix 10 cups of your favorite dry ingredients in a large bowl.

Use at least five cups of rolled oats. For the other five cups, add any combination of almonds, walnuts, pecans, cashews, coconut, raisins, dried cherries, dried dates, sunflower seeds, chia seeds, pumpkin seeds, ground flaxseed, ground chia seeds, organic wheat germ, quinoa, more oats, or any other dry ingredient you like. Stir the ingredients with a large spoon until thoroughly mixed.

Add your favorite spices.

Flavorful options include cinnamon, ginger, allspice, cloves, nutmeg. Stir with a large spoon until thoroughly mixed into the dry ingredients.

Mix 2 cups of liquid ingredients and pour over the dry ingredients.

Choose from raw local honey, olive oil, melted organic coconut oil, molasses, pure maple syrup or a combination of these.

Bake.

Choose any combination of ingredients you like. Just keep the proportions of dry and liquid the same: 10 cups of dry ingredients and 2 c of liquid ingredients.

This is one of my favorite combinations of ingredients.

In a large bowl mix the following dry ingredients:

5 cups of rolled steel cut oats

1 cup of quinoa

½ cup of milled ground flaxseed

½ cup raisins

1 cup chopped walnuts

1 cup chopped almonds

1 cup chopped or flaked unsweetened coconut. Look for a brand that contains only coconut with no added dyes and preservatives. Or coarsely chop fresh coconut.

1 tablespoon ground cinnamon

2 teaspoons of ground ginger

Mix the dry ingredients together until completely blended and set the bowl aside.

In a small pot heat on low until just about to boil:

1 ½ cups raw natural honey. Organic local honey is best.

3/4 cup olive oil

1/4 cup natural, nonhydrogenated organic coconut oil.

Stir the mixture as it heats. Remove the pot from the heat and add 1 tsp pure vanilla bean extract. Stir thoroughly.

Pour the heated mixture over the dry ingredients. Stir until all the dry ingredients are completely coated with the liquid. Spread the mixture out evenly onto three greased cookie sheets. Bake the sheets one at a time at 350 for 20 to 30 minutes. Stir half way through the cooking time. Let the granola cool on the cookie sheets. When it has completely cooled, break the mixture into small pieces. Store the granola in an airtight container. It will keep for six to eight weeks on your pantry shelf.

ENTREES

You can find thousands of recipes for main dishes and entrees in cookbooks and online to meet the needs of your family and your personal taste preferences. If you are used to always grabbing fast food or popping processed packaged dinners into the microwave, there are some simple strategies that make cooking an entree from scratch a snap.

Guidelines for Entrées
Follow the Ten Tips for Making Real Food Convenient listed at the beginning of the recipe section for entrées just as you would for any other meal course.

Start with a sensible portion of meat, poultry, or fish. We have normalized huge serving sizes due to routinely being served enough meat in restaurants in one dinner entrée to serve a family of four. One sensible serving of meat, poultry, or fish should be about the size of your palm.

Don't be afraid to experiment with ingredients. I rarely use recipes. I love to add a dash of this and a dollop of that.

Use foods and spices full of antioxidants and anti-inflammatory nutrients in every entrée you make. You'll notice some of the same ingredients are used in most of these main dishes. That's because they are full of nutrients that promote health and well-being. Refer back to the lists of real foods and spices in chapter nine for ideas.

Substitutions are allowed. In fact, they are so much fun that I highly recommend them. If you don't like a spice in one of the recipes, leave it out. If there is a spice you love that's not in the recipe, toss some of it into the pot.

Switch up the proteins. Many recipes will taste yummy no matter what you use for protein. Exchange shredded chicken for tuna or ground beef. Use sliced steak instead of sliced chicken to create a whole new dish.

Leave the meat out entirely. Try a vegetarian entrée for a change of pace and taste. Use cheese and eggs for protein instead of meat, fish or poultry.

Have fun creating meals from scratch. It's your house, your kitchen, your family, and your taste buds. Make what you like and if you don't like what you make, make something else the next time. Happy cooking!

Spicy Beef Stew

Preparing meals in a slow cooker is a good way to make sure you have a healthy dinner ready even on your busiest days. You can make this stew right after breakfast and let it cook all day while you are at work or busy running errands. If you are an Instant Pot fan, you can adapt this recipe (or any slow cooker recipe) for the times suggested in the owner's manual and throw this together after you get home in the afternoon. I prefer the slow cooker because I can do all the prep in the morning and have dinner ready to go at mealtime.

Put the following ingredients into a large slow cooker. Slow cookers come in different sizes. For this recipe you need to use one that holds at least six quarts.

1 pound of cubed beef stew meat. If possible, use beef from organically raised cows that contains no hormones or antibiotics. Cut the cubes into one-inch squares if the pieces are larger than this.

10 carrots cut into two-inch chunks. Wash the carrots thoroughly and peel with a vegetable peeler before chopping.

10 small red skin potatoes. Scrub the potatoes thoroughly but do not peel. Slice each potato into four chunks.

1 purple onion, peeled and finely chopped

4 cloves of garlic, peeled and finely chopped

2 stalks of celery, washed, scraped with a vegetable peeler, and finely chopped

2 whole tomatoes peeled and chopped into one-inch chunks. You can use one or two cans of chopped tomatoes instead of fresh, if you prefer. Be sure to read the label. Pick a brand that has fewer than five ingredients and does not contain added harmful chemicals such as BHT preservatives, MSG, or high fructose corn syrup.

You can add any other vegetables you like such as peas, beans, or corn.

Add:

1 spicy pepper: jalapeno, poblano, or cowhorn. Wash, seed, and chop the pepper. If you like super spicy food, toss in all three.

2 bay leaves

1 teaspoon ground cumin

1 teaspoon chili powder

1 teaspoon sea salt

1 teaspoon freshly ground pepper

1 tablespoon each of chopped fresh cilantro, basil, and oregano or ½ teaspoon each of these spices ground.

2 cans of beef broth. Read the labels and purchase a brand that has less than five ingredients with no added chemicals.

Add water so that there is enough total liquid in the pot to completely cover all of the ingredients.

Stir everything together until thoroughly mixed.

Cook on high for six hours or on low for eight to ten hours.

Change it up. Instead of 1 pound of cubed beef stew meat, use 1 pound of chicken or cooked ground chuck

Chicken Fajita Dinner

2 skinned, boneless chicken breasts cut into thin strips

1 small chopped purple onion

4 cloves of garlic peeled and finely minced

1 large red bell pepper cut into thin strips

1 large yellow bell pepper cut into thin strips

1 large green bell pepper cut into thin strips

10 button sized Portobello mushrooms, sliced

4 tablespoons of olive oil

Salt, pepper, chili powder, cilantro, cumin, turmeric to taste. Start with ¼ to ½ tsp. of each and adjust to your taste preference.

8 large whole wheat flour tortillas

Salsa

Cheese, grated sharp cheddar, mozzarella, or pepper jack

1 can of black beans with beans as the only ingredient listed on the label

2 cups of cooked whole grain rice

1 ripe avocado

In a large skillet or wok, sauté the first seven ingredients plus the spices you choose in the olive oil for five minutes or until the chicken is cooked all the way through.

Add ¼ cup of salsa to the beans and heat in a small pot.

I recommend cooking the rice in a rice cooker. It seals in the nutrients and comes out perfectly cooked every time.

To assemble dinner: Place a scoop of the cooked fajita mixture in the center of a flour tortilla. Top with a sprinkle of the grated cheese. Fold over two inches of the right side toward the middle. Fold over the long axis at the bottom and roll toward the top to create a handheld fajita. Serve with black beans, rice, and sliced avocado on the side.

Change it up. Instead of chicken, use ground beef, thinly sliced steak, or your favorite fish.

A Whole Lot of Chicken Goin' On

You can maximize your time by cooking food in large batches and freezing it to use later in a variety of recipes. Here's what you can do when you cook a large batch of chicken.

Buy 8 large boneless skinless chicken breasts. Put four of the breasts into a medium sized pot. Cut each of the remaining four chicken breasts into two filet pieces by slicing through the longest thickest side of each piece of chicken. If you have extra small bits of chicken leftover while slicing the breasts into filets, add them to the pot with the whole chicken breasts.

Put the 8 chicken fillets in a 9 x 13 glass baking dish. Make one of these marinades.

Basic Chicken Marinade

Mix in a small bowl using a wire whisk:

1 cup of olive oil

4 cloves of garlic, peeled and chopped

¼ cup purple onion, peeled and chopped

¼ teaspoon ground cilantro or 1 tablespoon fresh, chopped

¼ teaspoon cumin

¼ teaspoon rosemary or 1 tablespoon fresh, chopped

Honey Mustard Marinade

Start with the Basic Marinade Recipe.

Add 1 tablespoon of mustard and 4 tablespoons of raw organic honey to the mixture.

Mix with a wire whisk.

Ginger Lime Marinade

Start with the Basic Marinade Recipe.

Add 1 tablespoon of lime zest, the juice from 2 large limes, and 1 tablespoon of grated fresh gingerroot or ½ teaspoon ground ginger.

Mix with a wire whisk.

Change it up. Add your favorite spices and ingredients to the basic marinade recipe to create a whole new marinade.

Pour whichever marinade you choose to make over the 8 chicken fillets in the glass dish. Cover the dish and put it in the refrigerator to marinate overnight. You're going to grill the breasts tomorrow.

Now it's time to get back to the rest of the chicken you put in the large pot.

Add to the pot with the four other chicken breasts:

6 cloves of garlic, peeled and finely chopped

1 small purple or red onion, peeled and finely chopped.

1 teaspoon of ground cumin

1 teaspoon of cilantro or 1 tablespoon fresh, finely chopped

1 teaspoon of freshly ground pepper

1 teaspoon of sea salt

Add enough water to completely cover the chicken breasts. Bring the pot to a boil, and then reduce the heat to simmer. Simmer the chicken for 1 hour. Remove the chicken breasts and place on a plate to cool for 15 minutes. Shred the chicken into fine pieces using your fingers.

Divide the shredded chicken into one cup portions and put into freezer safe bags or containers. The total amount of shredded chicken you end up with will vary depending on the size of the chicken breasts you cooked. Label freezer containers with what is inside, the date you made it, and the number of servings. The shredded chicken is safely tucked away in your freezer ready to use in a wide variety of recipes.

The next day, remove the chicken filets from the marinade and grill on each side approximately five minutes or until there is no pink in the middle. Remove the grilled pieces of chicken to a plate to cool for 15 minutes. Place the grilled chicken filets into a freezer safe container with wax paper between the pieces of chicken. This will make it easier to remove the number of pieces of chicken you need without the pieces sticking together. The grilled chicken is now ready to grab and use in your favorite recipes.

BBQ Chicken Sandwiches

Defrost two cups of the shredded chicken. Do not defrost the cooked shredded chicken in the microwave if it is frozen in a plastic bag or container. Heating food in plastic containers can release harmful chemicals from the plastic that will leach into the food. Run hot water over the container for a couple of minutes to loosen the chicken from the container. Put it in a microwave safe glass bowl and heat in the microwave for one to two minutes to defrost.

Finely chop: ½ cup of green bell pepper, ½ cup of purple onion, 4 peeled garlic gloves.

Heat 2 tablespoon of olive oil in a large skillet over medium high heat.

Sautee the chopped vegetables in the oil for three minutes until they are translucent and just starting to brown.

Add the two cups of defrosted shredded chicken to the vegetables.

Add about 1 cup of your favorite organic bottled BBQ sauce. This will vary depending on how much liquid you prefer with BBQ. If you can't find organic BBQ sauce, choose a brand with the fewest added chemicals and count it as part of the 10% processed food you choose to use for that day. Or make your own BBQ sauce using the recipe below.

If you love spicy BBQ, add two shakes of Tabasco sauce and/ or 1chopped and seeded jalapeno, poblano, or cowhorn pepper.

Change it up. Instead of chicken, use thinly sliced steak or cooked ground chuck.

Serve over toasted buns. Makes 4 - 6 sandwiches.

Side dish: Prepared raw carrot and celery sticks described above. Just grab a handful and drain.

BBQ sauce

Note: If you can't find organic tomato sauce, ketchup and mustard, choose a brand with no added preservatives, artificial coloring, high fructose corn syrup, or other chemical additives.

1 large can organic tomato sauce. This will be about 15 oz., may vary according to brand.

1 cup of organic ketchup

½ cup organic mustard

½ cup apple cider vinegar

½ cup raw organic sugar

Juice from 3 lemons or limes

½ small purple onion, grated or finely chopped

½ teaspoon salt

1 teaspoon turmeric

½ teaspoon cayenne pepper

Mix all ingredients in a medium saucepan. Bring to a boil. Boil and stir until the mixture begins to thicken. Reduce to simmer and continue to cook and stir until it is the thickness you like.

Chicken Mushroom Burritos

Defrost two cups of shredded chicken.

In a large bowl mix: the defrosted chicken, 1 cup of sliced mushrooms, and 1 cup of salsa. Use prepared organic salsa, commercial salsa with the fewest added chemicals that you count toward your 10% processed food for the day, or make your own salsa using the recipe below.

Heat for three minutes on high in the microwave or for ten minutes over medium heat in a pot on the stove.

Put a scoop of the mixture in the center of a flour tortilla. Top with black olives and your favorite grated cheese. Fold over two inches of the right side toward the middle. Fold over the long axis at the bottom and roll toward the top to create a handheld burrito. Makes 4 - 6 burritos.

Note: Always grate your own cheese from a block of cheese. Packaged shredded cheese contains cellulose which is made from wood pulp. Who wants to eat sawdust with their cheese?

Change it up. Instead of chicken use cooked ground chuck, thinly sliced steak, or your favorite cooked fish.

Homemade Spicy Hot Salsa Recipe

2 cups chopped tomatoes

½ cup chopped purple onion

½ cup chopped green bell pepper, seeds and veins removed

4 cloves garlic, peeled and chopped

1 small jalapeno pepper, seeded and chopped

1 small can green chilies

Juice from 2 limes
1 teaspoon cilantro
1 teaspoon cumin
¼ teaspoon salt
¼ teaspoon cayenne pepper
¼ teaspoon turmeric

How do you like your salsa? Mild or spicy? Chunky or smooth? If you prefer a mild to medium salsa, leave out the jalapeno, cayenne, and/or green chilies. If you like smooth salsa, put all ingredients in a food processor and blend until it is the consistency you prefer. If you like chunky salsa, set half of the chopped vegetables aside and blend the other half plus the spices in a food processor and then add the reserved chopped vegetables. Homemade salsa tastes best when used immediately. It will keep in the refrigerator in a tightly covered container for several days. Throw the leftovers away if you haven't used it all within one week. If you make a recipe that calls for salsa and eat the rest with tortilla chips, it will be gone in a day. And yes, you can eat commercially made tortilla chips. Choose a brand with the fewest ingredients and count it toward your 10% processed food for the day. The brand I eat contains only three ingredients: corn, vegetable oil, and salt.

Side dish: Black beans and rice. Cook one cup of rice in a rice cooker. Add 1 teaspoon of cumin and 1 teaspoon of chili powder to one can of black beans that has only one ingredient: the beans. Do not drain the beans. Heat in a small pan over medium heat until hot and bubbly. For each serving put ½ cup cooked rice on the plate topped with ¼ cup black beans. Sprinkle with ½ teaspoon of cilantro.

Chicken Salad

The day before you plan to make the salad, take 2 cups of shredded chicken out of the freezer and put in the refrigerator to defrost overnight.

In a large mixing bowl put:

2 cups defrosted shredded chicken

½ cup of finely chopped walnuts, pecans, or almonds or a mixture of all three.

½ cup dill pickle relish, thoroughly drained. Note: If the relish contains artificial food coloring, preservatives, etc. count this as part of your 10% processed food for the day.

In a small bowl mix with a wire whisk:

½ cup organic mayonnaise

¼ cup organic mustard

½ teaspoon salt

½ teaspoon cumin

½ teaspoon cilantro

½ teaspoon rosemary

¼ teaspoon turmeric

¼ teaspoon cayenne pepper

Pour the sauce mixture over the chicken mixture. Stir until well blended. Chill for at least one hour. Serve the chicken salad on toasted bread or put a scoop on a bed of mixed salad greens. If you are taking the chicken salad to a party, put it into your favorite glass serving dish. Sprinkle the top with finely chopped nuts or cut grapes into halves and arrange them in a pretty design on top of the salad.

Change it up. Use 2 cups of flaked white tuna in place of the shredded chicken.

Chicken Pot Pie

2 cups defrosted shredded chicken

3 large baking potatoes, peeled and chopped into 2-inch chunks

1 large package of frozen peas and carrots that contains only two ingredients: peas and carrots

½ small purple onion, peeled and finely chopped

4 garlic cloves, peeled and finely chopped

3 cups of chicken broth. Save the broth from boiling the chicken or buy canned broth that has no added chemical ingredients.

Milk

2 tablespoons butter

2 tablespoons olive oil

4 tablespoons unbleached all-purpose flour

1 teaspoon cumin

1 teaspoon cilantro

½ teaspoon turmeric

1 teaspoon of salt

Ground pepper, two twists of pepper grinder or to taste

If you love everything spicy, add a dash of hot sauce and/or ½ teaspoon of cayenne pepper.

1 pie crust. Use your favorite pie crust recipe or purchase a premade crust that you can roll out. If you use the premade crust, count it toward your 10 % processed food for the day

Grease a 9 x 13 pan with butter and set aside.

Put the broth in a large pot and bring to a boil. Add the chopped onion, garlic, and potatoes and cook over medium heat keeping the liquid at a gentle boil for 15 - 20 minutes or until the potatoes are tender. If you can stick a fork easily into the potato pieces, they are ready.

Add the frozen peas and carrots and cook for an additional 8 - 10 minutes or until tender.

Drain the vegetables and save the broth. Mix the cooked vegetables with the shredded chicken and put in the greased 9 x 13 pan.

Measure the broth in a large glass 4 cup or larger measuring cup. Some broth may evaporate while you are cooking the vegetables. If you do not have 3 cups of broth left, add enough milk to make 3 cups total of liquid.

In a large skillet, heat the butter and olive oil over medium high heat until the butter is melted and the mixture is sizzling. Reduce the heat to medium low. Sprinkle the flour over the melted butter and oil mixture and stir constantly with a wire whisk. Cook the mixture for about 3 minutes or until the flour is completely incorporated and is just starting to turn a golden brown. Slowly add the liquid broth/milk mixture to the skillet and continue to stir. Stir until the mixture starts to thicken and then remove from the heat. Note: Sauces can be a little tricky if you've never tried to make them from scratch before. But they can nearly always be rescued. The first time I made this, I added the flour while the skillet was too hot and it clumped up into a thick mess. I just added the liquid and kept stirring and it smoothed out and all was well.

After you remove the skillet from the heat, add the salt, pepper, and spices and thoroughly mix. Pour the sauce over the chicken and vegetable mixture in the pan.

Roll out the homemade or premade pie crust onto a floured cutting board. Cut the crust into strips. Place half of the strips across the width of the pan and half across the length to create a lattice like crust.

Use a pastry brush to brush the top of the crust with a little milk.

Bake the chicken pie in the preheated oven for 45 - 60 minutes until the mixture is hot and bubbly and the crust is golden brown.

Serve with fresh fruit.

Divide the leftovers into single serving portions and freeze for later.

Chicken Pasta Marinara

Note: If you can't find organic canned tomatoes and tomato sauce, choose a brand with the fewest chemical ingredients and count it toward your 10% processed food for the day.

1 can whole organic tomatoes

1 can organic tomato sauce

1 teaspoon ground oregano

½ teaspoon ground basil

½ teaspoon freshly ground black pepper

½ teaspoon ground turmeric

¼ teaspoon ground cayenne pepper

½ purple or yellow onion, peeled and finely chopped

4 cloves garlic, peeled and finely chopped

3 tablespoons olive oil

2 defrosted grilled chicken breasts, sliced into thin finger sized pieces.

Your favorite pasta, enough for 4 servings. I like to use vermicelli for this dish, but you can use any kind of pasta and it will be delish

Parmesan cheese

Fresh parsley, finely chopped. If you can't find fresh, grab a jar of dried parsley in the spice section of your favorite supermarket.

Put the tomatoes, tomato sauce, and all the spices into a blender or food processor. Pulse until everything is blended and the tomatoes are in little pieces.

Sautee the chopped onion and garlic in the olive oil in a large heavy saucepan over medium heat. Add the pureed tomato sauce and spices and mix well. Simmer over low heat for 1 hr.

Cook 4 servings of your favorite pasta according to the directions on the package.

Put the defrosted chicken in a microwave safe bowl and microwave on high for 1 minute until completely warmed through.

To assemble:

Put a serving of pasta on a pretty plate.

Spoon sauce over the pasta.

Arrange ¼ of the thinly sliced grilled chicken pieces in a fan shape on top of the sauce.

Sprinkle with parmesan cheese.

Sprinkle fresh or dried parsley over the top.

Serve with toasted garlic bread and a side salad.

Change it up. Instead of chicken, use cooked ground chuck, thinly sliced cooked beef, or your favorite fish or seafood.

Grilled Chicken with Avocado Sandwiches

2 cooked frozen grilled chicken breasts that you prepared earlier, defrosted.

2 toasted whole grain sandwich buns

1 ripe avocado peeled and sliced

Juice from 1 lime

Spicy mustard

Mixed salad greens

1 ripe tomato, sliced

Sprinkle the chicken breasts with 1tablespoon of water, cover, and warm in the microwave until just warmed through. Do not overheat as this will make the chicken dry.

Spread spicy mustard over both halves of the bun.

Layer each sandwich in this order: grilled chicken, tomato, salad greens, avocado slices. Squeeze a fresh lime over the avocado pieces letting some of the juice drip down over the salad greens.

Serve with carrot and celery sticks and your favorite fresh fruit on the side.

Change it up. Instead of grilled chicken, use grilled steak or grilled salmon.

Asian Stir-Fried Chicken

4 cups of cooked rice.

1 frozen grilled chicken breast, defrosted and cut into bite sized slivers.

1 small purple onion, peeled and finely chopped

6 garlic cloves, peeled and finely chopped

1 cup of your favorite vegetables finely chopped. You can use fresh veggies, cooked leftovers, or frozen vegetables. If you use fresh vegetables, chop them extra fine or grate them so that they will cook more quickly. Choose from carrots, cauliflower, broccoli, any color of bell peppers, green beans, or any other vegetable you like.

1 cup of thinly sliced white button or baby portobello mushrooms

6 tablespoons of olive oil

1 teaspoon salt

1teaspoon freshly ground black pepper

½ teaspoon red cayenne pepper

½ teaspoon turmeric

½ teaspoon ground cumin

½ teaspoon cilantro

2 beaten eggs. Use free-range organic eggs, if possible.

Parsley, freshly chopped or dried.

Heat the olive oil in a large wok. If you don't have a wok, use a large heavy saucepot or Dutch oven.

Add the chopped onion and garlic and the fresh vegetables, if you are using fresh. If you are using leftover or frozen vegetables, don't add them yet.

Cook and stir over the sizzling heat for 2 to 5 minutes or until the onion and garlic start to brown.

Add the sliced mushrooms. If you use leftover or frozen vegetables, add them with the mushrooms.

Keep the heat on medium high and cook and stir for 3 minutes.

Add the rice and the defrosted sliced chicken. Sprinkle in all the seasonings. Stir so that the vegetables and spices are mixed in well and the rice and chicken are completely covered with oil.

Stir and cook for 5 minutes over the sizzling heat.

Reduce the temperature to medium low.

Pour the beaten eggs over the top of the mixture. Stir the eggs in carefully with a spoon, tossing and gently stirring the mixture for 5 minutes until you see small bits of cooked egg throughout the mixture.

Serve piping hot sprinkled with parsley. Add a fresh green side salad or a fruit salad and serve with warm toasted flatbread triangles.

Change it up. Instead of chicken, use thinly sliced steak or your favorite fish.

Chicken Loaded Baked Potatoes

4 medium sized Idaho baking potatoes
4 grilled chicken fingers, defrosted
Butter
Grated cheese
Black olives
1 avocado, peeled and sliced
Sour cream
Salsa
Sea salt
Freshly ground black pepper
Favorite spices

To get the flavor and texture of an oven baked potato in a fraction of the time, preheat the oven to 450. Scrub the potatoes under running water. Pat dry with a paper towel. Poke a fork into each potato about 20 times turning potato as you go to make sure it is poked with the fork on all sides.

Place the potatoes on a microwave safe plate or dish. Cook the potatoes on high in the microwave for 18 minutes. Use an oven mitt to gently squeeze the potatoes to see if they feel soft. If they still feel hard, cook for 6 more minutes and check again.

When the potatoes feel soft, they are done. Transfer them to a metal pan and put them in the preheated oven. Leave in the oven for 15 minutes. This will make the potatoes fluff up just like they do when baked in the oven for a couple of hours.

Heat the chicken fingers in the microwave for 1 minute or until hot. Do not overcook or they will be too tough to chew. Cut each finger into bite sized pieces.

Cut each baked potato in half.

Top each potato with butter, salt, pepper, one cut up cooked chicken finger, your favorite spices, and any or all of the other toppings on the ingredients list.

Change it up. Use cooked ground chuck or thin slivers of grilled steak instead of the chicken. Cook extra potatoes and freeze them to use later. To reheat. Put 1 frozen potato on a microwave safe plate. Heat for 2 minutes on high. If the potato isn't hot enough, continue to heat in 30 second increments until it is heated through. Do not overheat as this will make the potato tough.

You can cook other meats in large batches and use it for multiple recipes like you did with the chicken. Here are a few ideas for ground beef and roast beef to get you started.

Cook a Bunch of Beef

Buy two large packages of ground chuck. Make hamburger patties out of one package and cook on the grill. Put the cooked hamburger patties into a labeled freezer-safe container between layers of wax paper. To serve: remove one hamburger patty. Heat the frozen patty in the microwave for one minute and serve on a bun to have a hamburger for a quick lunch. Make a sauce out of chopped garlic and sliced mushrooms sautéed in olive oil to pour over the patty and use it as the entrée for a meal. Add a baked sweet potato and some steamed or roasted broccoli and you have a delicious dinner and sides ready in no time.

Cook the other package of ground chuck by scrambling and stirring in a large skillet. Freeze the scrambled cooked ground chuck in 1 cup portions in a freezer safe container. Take it out as needed to make spaghetti sauce, nachos grandes, sloppy joes, chili, or any other dish that requires cooked scrambled ground beef. Substitute ground turkey for the hamburger meat for an even healthier choice. If you have never used ground turkey before, try making the patties out of half hamburger and half turkey or cooking half scrambled ground beef and half scrambled turkey. Either combination will taste like the hamburger meat you are used to but be healthier with the addition of turkey which is a much leaner meat.

Slow Cooker Pot Roast

Slow cookers and Instant Pots are a big help in preparing real food meals and avoiding processed food. Follow manufacturer directions to make this is your specific appliance. Here's how to make it in a slow cooker. Place in a slow cooker 3 peeled and chopped potatoes, 6 sliced carrots, ½ of a chopped red or purple onion, 4 gloves of chopped garlic. Place a 4-pound chuck or rump roast on top of the vegetables. If you want to splurge, use a sirloin tip roast. Season the roast with freshly ground pepper, sea salt, and your favorite herbs and spices. I like to add freshly chopped oregano that I grow on my deck in the summer. Pour a can of no added MSG beef broth over the roast. Cook in the slow cooker on high for six hours. Add a side salad or some fruit and you have a complete dinner ready on the day you cook the roast. Put leftover roast and vegetables into labeled freezer safe containers to have a frozen dinner that you created yourself. Put slices of beef without the vegetables in labeled freezer safe containers to use for roast beef sandwiches.

FUN WITH FRUIT

Pineapple, grapes, oranges, strawberries, kiwi, bananas, apples, and many other fruits are wonderful sources of antioxidants and anti-inflammatory nutrients. Keeping fruit in a pretty container on your counter or in your fridge makes it easy for you to grab something healthy for meals and snacks throughout the day.

Artistic Fruit Plates

If you are asked to bring a dish to a family gathering or neighborhood potluck dinner, volunteer to bring a fruit plate. This will assure that you have a healthy real food choice at the meal. There are many creative ways to arrange fruit that will make your fruit plate a standout dish.

Arrange the fruit in an abstract pattern alternating colors and textures. Create a butterfly by outlining the wings with grapes, putting a row of kiwi in the center for the body, and filling in the design with orange slices and bananas. Arrange the fruit to look like a flower. Use different kinds of fruit to form a stem, leaves, and flower petals. For a children's party arrange the fruit to form a face or a favorite animal.

Fruit Smoothies

For a basic smoothie: Crush 12 ice cubes in a blender.

Add ½ of a banana, ½ cup of almond milk, ½ tsp. of vanilla extract, and 2 tablespoons of raw organic honey.

Blend until the smoothie is the consistency you like. Add a little more almond milk if you want a thinner smoothie. Add another ice cube or two if you want your smoothie to be thicker.

There are all kinds of flavor variations you can make by adding ingredients to the basic smoothie recipe. Add a handful of strawberries, blueberries, or raspberries or a combination of your favorite berries. Add a small peach, peeled and cut into chunks for a yummy peach smoothie. Add tablespoons of raw cocoa powder and 2 tablespoons of creamy almond butter for a delicious chocolate almond smoothie.

Ginger

Ginger is one of my favorite anti-inflammatory foods. I toss it in stir-fry recipes, add it to bread, and drink a cup of ginger tea every morning with breakfast.

Ginger Tea

Ginger tea is one of my very favorite things to make that is full of antioxidants and anti-inflammatory ingredients. I drink a large cup every morning with breakfast and often have another cup at night. I use tea with caffeine in the mornings but only use decaffeinated tea after midday so that my sleep pattern will stay on track. When I first started making the ginger tea, I drank at least three cups a day every day for several weeks to reduce inflammation and help jumpstart the healing process.

Peel a one to two-inch slice of fresh ginger root.

Use a microplane grater to finely grate 1 tablespoon of the fresh ginger. You may want to make your first cup of ginger tea using 1 teaspoon rather than 1 tablespoon and increase the amount of ginger a little bit each day until you get used to the taste of the ginger. It is quite spicy.

You can use any mug you have and any type of tea that comes in a tea bag. Or you can use an infuser mug and your favorite organic loose-leaf tea.

If you are using a regular mug and tea bag, put the grated ginger into the mug.

Add 1 to 2 teaspoon of raw local honey.

Add the juice from one slice of lime or lemon.

Add 1/4 teaspoon of ground cinnamon.

Wait for the teakettle to whistle.

Fill the mug half full with boiling water.

Stir briskly to thoroughly mix the ingredients and dissolve the ginger.

Add a single serving size tea bag of your favorite black or green tea. Add hot water to finish filling up the mug.

Steep the tea for three to five minutes depending on how strong you like your tea.

Remove the tea bag and enjoy.

I like to use an infuser tea mug that has an inner removable strainer and use loose leaf organic tea. If you use an infuser mug, put the grated ginger and your favorite loose leaf organic tea into the infuser. Oolong, Darjeeling, and Irish Breakfast are some of my favorite loose leaf organic teas. Add a slice of lime or lemon and hot water boiled in a teakettle. After the tea has steeped for 4 minutes, remove the inner infuser liner and add the honey and cinnamon. Stir and enjoy.

Tips for Using and Storing Fresh Ginger
If you are not accustomed to using fresh ginger here are some tips to get you started.

Buy a microplane grater. It is a must have tool for grating fresh ginger to the right consistency so that it will dissolve in the tea or mix well with any recipes that call for fresh ginger.

Peel only the amount of ginger you need for making one cup of tea.

Never store fresh ginger in plastic containers or plastic wrap.

Put unused ginger into a plain brown paper lunch bag.

Store the ginger in the refrigerator.

Wrap the cut end of ginger in waxed paper before putting it back into the paper bag.

Once you become comfortable with using freshly grated ginger, there are a variety of other recipes you may want to try. Ginger adds a wonderful flavor to stir fry foods, salads, muffins, and cookies.

SALTY SNACKS

Salty snack foods are a processed food that almost everyone is used to buying and consuming. If you continue to buy processed chips, look for brands that have less than five ingredients and have no preservatives or dyes. If you want to experiment making your own, here are some ideas. Do you adore scrumptious chips? Try one of these.

Baked Pita Chips

Ingredients:

1 package of whole wheat pita bread with no additives

Olive oil

Your favorite spices

Directions:

Brush the whole pita rounds with olive oil.

Cut each pita round into 8 triangles.

Place the triangles on a cookie sheet that has been brushed with olive oil

Sprinkle the pita triangles with your favorite spices: garlic salt, onion powder, pepper, chili powder, cumin, cilantro, parsley, basil, oregano, ground pepper, sea salt. Pick one spice or sprinkle with a combination of your favorites.

Bake at 350 degrees until the chips turn light brown. Oven temperatures vary. This should take about 15 minutes. Serve warm with your favorite dip. Store the leftovers in an airtight container for future snacking. They will stay fresh and crispy for up to one week.

Baked Potato Chips

Ingredients:
    One to two russet potatoes
    3 tablespoons olive oil
    Sea salt
    Freshly ground black pepper.
    Use a mandoline to cut the potatoes into 1/16" slices. You can cut the potatoes with a sharp knife but a mandoline will produce uniform thin slices that result in a crunchy delicious potato chip.
    Brush a cookie sheet with olive oil.
    Lay the potato slices in a single layer on the cookie sheet.
    Brush the tops of the potatoes with olive oil.
    Sprinkle with salt and pepper.
    You can also sprinkle with your favorite spices.
    Bake at 450 degrees for 15 minutes until they are golden brown
    Remove from cookie sheet to a plate lined with paper towels
    Drain off excess oil.
    Serve warm or at room temperature.
    I recommend cooking only one batch of chips at a time. The chips are better if you eat them immediately after cooking instead of trying to store them to eat later.

Sweet Potato Chips

Follow the instructions for potato chips substituting two sweet potatoes for the russet potatoes for a delicious nutritious snack. The sweet potato chips are delicious sprinkled with garlic salt and pepper. For a sweeter version, sprinkle with salt, cinnamon, ground ginger, and a dusting of brown sugar.

Zucchini Chips

Use thinly sliced unpeeled zucchini instead of potatoes. Season with your favorite spices. I like to use spices with a little kick for these like chili powder, turmeric, and cumin. Brush with olive oil and follow the baking instructions above.

If popcorn is more your thing than chips, this recipe is delicious and easy.

Microwave Popcorn in a Brown Bag

This is my favorite salty snack discovery. Microwave popcorn is so convenient. When I read the ingredients label on the package, I found out it is also a huge source of chemical contamination. So, I make this instead. You only need a few simple things to make a delicious salty treat.

Buy a jar of GMO-free organic popcorn.

Get a package of small brown paper lunch bags.

To make the popcorn:

Put ¼ cup of popcorn in the lunch bag.

Fold the top of the bag over 1" and make a crease. Continue folding over 1" and creasing until you get to the popcorn at the bottom of the bag.

Put the bag in the microwave. Microwave ovens vary so you will have to test to determine the perfect timing for your oven. Mine takes 1 minute and 45 seconds to cook. Start with three minutes. Listen for the kernels to start popping. As the kernels pop the folds and creases you made in the bag will unroll. The sound of popping will increase and then start to slow. When the popping sound slows down take the bag out of the microwave.

Pour the popcorn into a large bowl. Drizzle with melted butter, sprinkle with a little salt, toss to coat, and dive into the deliciousness.

SWEET TREATS

When I created strategies for healthy living, I wanted them to be practical and easy to integrate into my daily routine. I have an incredible sweet tooth. So, completely eliminating sweets didn't seem very practical. I found a way to include sweet treats in my diet without blowing the healthy eating part of my plan. Eating a lot of refined sugar can trigger increased inflammation in your body that leads to all kinds of diseases. I don't eat an excessive amount of sugar, but I haven't eliminated it all together either. I have four guidelines for adding sweet treats to my healthy eating plan:

I eat real whole food for at least 90% of my diet every day. The other 10% is flexible. It includes occasional processed food with 5 ingredients or less, eating out when I'm not sure of the ingredients used in the food, and sweet treats.

I can eat whatever sweet treat I want as long as I make it myself from real food ingredients. This accomplishes two things: I know exactly what is in the food and I don't eat it nearly as often as I would if I grabbed a package or box of something from the grocery store. (Boxes of cake mix, bowls of whipped topping, packages of cookies aren't real food ingredients. I was amazed how many of my old "from scratch" baking recipes involved dumping various processed foods together.)

I substitute healthier ingredients for less healthy ones.

I add healthy ingredients to everything I bake to increase the nutritional value.

Easy recipe substitutions:

coconut oil or olive oil instead of vegetable oils and shortening

raw organic sugar, organic honey, real molasses, or real maple syrup instead of highly refined white sugar

whole wheat flour instead of refined white flour

Healthy ingredients that are easily added to sweet treats:

dried fruit
fresh fruit
ground milled flaxseed and ground chia seeds
nuts
nut butters
oatmeal
whole seeds like pumpkin seeds and sunflower seeds

I was a world class sugar addict before I started eating foods that promote healing. If you have a sweet tooth, it is important to find recipes that will satisfy your craving for a sweet snack but also have a higher nutritional value and do not expose you to the toxic chemicals used in commercially produced cookies and candy.

Some health experts recommend completely eliminating sugar from your diet. For me, that was not a practical plan. Limiting my sugar intake was a more attainable goal than cutting out sweets all together.

I stopped eating processed sugary foods. I no longer eat packaged candy and cookies. I eliminated things that contain high fructose corn syrup. I love to bake but now I bake only occasionally instead of all the time. I no longer bake things that call for large amounts of highly processed white refined sugar. I use raw organic cane sugar, organic brown sugar, molasses, pure maple syrup, or raw local honey in recipes. I try to make sure everything I bake includes nutritional ingredients. If I make a batch of cookies or brownies, I put them in the freezer and defrost only one at a time. This helps me with portion control. If I left a plate of cookies on the counter, I could polish them off all by myself in a day.

Here are a few sweet treat recipes.

GBJ's Brownies

My whole family adores my mother's brownie recipe. We have been eating Grandmother Betty Jo's brownies for four generations. However, the original recipe contains some ingredients that I no longer eat such as shortening, refined white flour, and refined white sugar. I have adapted the recipe to fit my healthy living plan and am still able to keep the family tradition alive. I have made healthier substitutions for the shortening originally called for and I add nuts and flaxseed to up the nutritional value. Brownies are by no stretch of the imagination a health food. However, I have found that you can take almost any recipe and change a few ingredients here and there to make it a little healthier. These brownies are quite sweet. To limit my daily sugar intake, I usually eat no more than one per day and I don't eat them every day. I make them only when the grandchildren are in town for a visit or for other special occasions. (Such as it's a random Tuesday in July and I'm craving brownies).

Preheat the oven to 350.

In a large mixing bowl stir together until well blended:

1 cup of unbleached flour

½ cup of whole wheat flour. For a gluten free version, use coconut, rice, tapioca, or almond flour or a mixture of these gluten free flours in place of the unbleached white flour and wheat flour.

1 ½ cups of raw organic sugar. The original recipe called for 2 cups of refined white sugar but they are still quite sweet with the lesser amount.

2 tablespoons of ground milled flaxseed or a combination of ground flaxseed and ground chia seed

2/3 cup of raw cocoa powder with no additives

1 teaspoon salt

To this mixture add and beat well with an electric mixer:

4 eggs. Use organic free-range eggs when available.

2 teaspoons of pure vanilla extract

The original recipe called for 1 cup of shortening which is full of hydrogenated trans fats. Instead use:

1/3 cup olive oil

1/3 cup solid organic non-hydrogenated coconut oil

1/3 cup butter (or butter substitute if you prefer dairy free)

Beat with an electric mixer until thoroughly mixed.

Add 1 cup of chopped walnuts, almonds, or pecans or a mixture of the three nuts.

Place mixture in a greased 9 x 13 metal pan and smooth out with a spatula.

Bake at 350 for 25 to 30 minutes until there is no sheen left on the top and the edges are starting to brown and pull away from the sides of the pan.

Let the brownies completely cool in the pan. Cut into 40 bars. The original recipe said to cut into 24 bars. Making smaller serving sizes is a good way to enjoy a sweet treat in moderation.

Two in One Oatmeal Cookies

Love cookies? Two in One Oatmeal Cookies are delicious and full of healthy ingredients. They are a time saver because you can make two different kinds of cookies out of the same batch of batter: Raisin Nut Oatmeal Cookies and Chocolate Chip Oatmeal Cookies.

You can make a gluten free version of these cookies by using 2 cups of gluten free flour such as coconut flour, rice flour, tapioca flour, and/or almond flour in place of the unbleached flour and the whole wheat flour.

You can make them dairy free by using almond milk and a dairy free butter substitute in place of the milk and butter.

You can substitute peanut butter for the almond butter. If you do, buy a brand of natural peanut butter that only contains peanuts and a little salt. Many commercial brands of peanut butter contain added ingredients including high fructose corn syrup, soy, sugar, and hydrogenated oils full of harmful trans fats. I prefer almond butter because it has more nutritional value than peanut butter. Peanuts cause an increased inflammatory response in some folks and almonds are an anti-inflammatory food. Almond butter contains omega 3 and omega 6 fatty acids, niacin, folate, calcium, iron, riboflavin, manganese, and other healthy minerals. Look for an organic brand that contains fewer than five ingredients.

Preheat the oven to 325.

Cream together in a large mixing bowl using an electric mixer:

1/3 cup of organic coconut oil

1/3 cup of butter, or butter substitute if you want them to be dairy free

1/3 cup of almond butter

1/4 cup raw honey

1/2 cup raw organic sugar

3/4 cup raw organic brown sugar

Beat in:

2 eggs, use organic free-range eggs when possible

2 teaspoons of pure vanilla extract

1/3 cup milk. Use almond milk if you want them to be dairy free.

In a separate bowl mix together:

1 cup unbleached flour

1 cup of whole wheat flour.

½ teaspoon baking soda

½ teaspoon salt

1 tablespoon of milled flaxseed or ground flaxseed and chia seed combo.

4 cups of rolled oats, regular not quick cooking

Blend the flour mixture thoroughly into the creamed mixture.

Scoop out half the batter into another mixing bowl. This will be approximately 2 ½ cups of batter.

Add 1 cup of chocolate chips to this bowl. I use Enjoy Life Mini Chocolate Chips. They are dairy free, gluten free, soy free, and peanut free.

Stir with a large spoon until the chocolate chips are completely blended into the batter.

Set this bowl aside.

To the batter in the other bowl add:

½ cup chopped walnuts

½ cup chopped almonds

½ cup raisins

½ teaspoon ground cinnamon

½ teaspoon ground ginger

Mix with an electric mixer until all of the ingredients are completely blended.

For each cookie, scoop out 1 heaping tablespoon of dough. Put the ball of dough onto a greased cookie sheet. Leave 1" of space between each cookie. Flatten the cookie balls slightly with your hand, the back of a spoon, or a spatula. Grease whatever you use (including your hand) with a little butter or oil so the dough won't stick when you flatten the cookies.

Bake at 325 for 11 to 14 minutes or until the cookies are lightly browned on the bottom and just starting to turn a golden brown on the top.

Remove the cookie sheet from the oven and allow the cookies to cool for 2 minutes on the cookie sheet. Use a spatula to remove the cookies from the cookie sheet and place on a wire rack to cool completely. This recipe makes about 80 cookies, 40 of each kind. Store them in an airtight container if you are planning to serve them within a couple of days. Store them in a freezer safe container or bag if you want to bake them ahead of time to serve later. I like to freeze them and take out a couple at a time when I'm in the mood for a little sweet treat. Microwave two cookies for about 20 seconds for a warm treat or take as many as you need out of the freezer and leave at room temperature to defrost if you want to serve a plateful at a family gathering or party.

Holiday Baking

We have a lot of family recipes that several generations have enjoyed eating during the Thanksgiving and Christmas holidays. I have learned to bake versions of these family favorites that are healthier than the original recipes so that we can continue our family traditions.

We have baked cutout and decorated Christmas sugar cookies every year since my children were small and now enjoy baking them with our grandchildren. It was an exercise in creativity to decide how to continue the tradition without using chemically laden ingredients. I didn't want to use commercially made food coloring because it is made out of petroleum products that are toxic. I wanted my grandchildren to have fun making the cookies I had made with my children. The sugar cookies we ended up making are a great example of how you can adapt almost any recipe if you are willing to be flexible and try a creative challenge. Christmas is one occasion where I am a little more flexible about using sugar. I am still able to stick to my rule of making sure that 90% of what I consume is healthy whole foods and having a little more leeway with the remaining 10% of what I eat.

Iced Cutout Christmas Sugar Cookies

Mix together:

3 cups of unbleached white flour. For a gluten free version substitute 1 cup of white rice flour,1 cup of tapioca flour, and 1 cup of almond flour.

½ teaspoon baking powder

½ teaspoon salt

Add:

1 cup of chilled unsalted butter. For a dairy free version, use 2/3 cup of organic butter substitute and 1/3 cup of nonhydrogenated organic coconut oil.

Cut this into the flour mixture using a pastry blender until well blended

Add:

1 egg

4 tablespoons of milk. Use almond milk for a dairy free version.

1 teaspoon of pure vanilla extract.

Begin by stirring this in with a spoon. Finish by kneading all of the ingredients together with your hands until you can form a smooth ball of dough that sticks together. If the dough seems too dry, add milk a little at a time until you can make a smooth ball of dough. If the dough seems too sticky, add a little flour at a time until you can form a smooth ball of dough.

Cover the dough and refrigerate for at least one hour or overnight. I make the dough and refrigerate it overnight the day before we plan to make the cookies.

Pinch off about 1/3 cup of dough at a time and use a rolling pin to roll out the dough about ¼ inch thick on a floured cutting board. Cut out desired shapes with cookie cutters. Put leftover dough back into the bowl and use your hands to knead it back into the chilled dough ball. Use a spatula to transfer the cookies to a greased cookie sheet.

Bake at 400 for 8 minutes. Remove the cookie sheet from the oven. Let the cookies cool on the sheet for 2 minutes and then remove with a spatula and place on a cooling rack. Completely cool the cookies before icing.

Icing: Mix 1 box of confectioner sugar, 1 teaspoon of pure vanilla extract, ½ cup of butter or butter substitute, and 2 tablespoons of milk or almond milk with an electric mixer. Add a little more confectioner sugar if the mixture seems too thin. Add a little more milk if it seems too thick.

Divide the icing into several small bowls. Add homemade food coloring to the bowls and stir. Leave one bowl white. Use the icing to decorate the cookies however you want.

Food coloring is a harmful chemical additive made out of petroleum derivatives. If you do not have time to make your own food coloring, use only a small drop of the commercially produced coloring or ice the cookies with uncolored frosting. There are many ways to make your own food coloring using natural products. All of these colors are pastels. You can get deeper colors by adding more of the homemade coloring but the liquid will change the consistency of the icing so you will have to adjust the recipe measurements. Note: To save time, I made the fruit-based food colorings described below the week before my family came to visit and froze in small containers. I moved the containers from the freezer to the refrigerator to defrost the day before we made the cookies.

Pink. Puree fresh strawberries in a blender. Pour through a strainer so that you only have juice and no pulp left. Cook in a small pan over low heat until the liquid is reduced to about 1/4 of what you started out with. Refrigerate or freeze for later use. Besides turning the icing a lovely shade of pink, you get a nice strawberry flavor.

Purple. Use fresh or frozen blueberries and repeat the steps as listed for the pink strawberry color above.

Blue. Make the purple coloring using the blueberries as described above. Add a small pinch of baking soda to the reduced blueberry liquid. It will start changing to a blue color. Keep adding small pinches of baking soda until it is the shade of blue that you want.

Brown. Add cinnamon to the icing until you get the shade of brown you want. This will add a nice light spicy cinnamon flavor to the icing.

You can also add fruit juices to the icing to get the color you want. Try cranberry, grape, and orange juice. Make sure the juice contains 100 % juice with no added sugar or high fructose corn syrup.

VEGETABLES

Roasted Vegetables

Broccoli, cabbage, cauliflower, garlic, onions, red skinned potatoes, squash, and zucchini are delicious roasted in the oven. This is a simple side dish to prepare.

Preheat the oven to 450 degrees.

Brush a rimmed cookie sheet with olive oil.

Place cut up vegetables on the cookie sheet.

Brush the vegetables with olive oil.

Sprinkle with sea salt and freshly ground black pepper.

Bake for 30 minutes to one hour or until the vegetables are tender and beginning to brown around the edges. The cooking time will vary depending on which vegetables you choose.

Serve hot.

COOKING FOR THE ALLERGY CROWD: DAIRY FREE, GLUTEN FREE, PEANUT FREE IDEAS

My extended family has food allergies or food sensitivities to many different kinds of foods including dairy, peanuts, gluten, and soy. I have experimented and found ways to adapt many recipes to meet our food challenges.

Here are some simple substitutions.

Butter. There are various butter substitutes on the market. My favorite is the soy free version of Earth Balance Butter Substitute. It works well for baking, sautéing, and spreading.

This is not ideal as butter substitutes contain some ingredients I would prefer not to consume. However, it meets my goal of practicality and since I only use it for special occasions, I stay within my 90% real food goal. In some recipes I am able to substitute organic coconut oil or olive oil for the butter. These are more natural choices.

Wheat Flour. I do not like to use prepackaged gluten free flour because of the xanthan gum, guar gum and other additives commonly used in the production process. There are many kinds of gluten free flour available including coconut, almond, rice, tapioca, sorghum, and quinoa flours that have no additives. Different flours work best for different recipes. I like to use a mixture of about half white rice flour and half tapioca flour with a few tablespoons of almond and sorghum flour for most recipes. There are things you can do to make up for the binding and rising qualities found in gluten. I mix one tablespoon of ground flax seed with two tablespoons of boiling water and add to recipes for baked items like breads, cake, and cookies. Adding an extra egg to your favorite recipe and separating the eggs will help with the texture of gluten free baked foods. Beat the whites until stiff and fold in last to add some moisture and a little lift. Add ½ to 1 teaspoon more baking powder than your recipe calls for to help make up for the rising power of gluten.

Milk. In place of milk, I use almond milk. Look for a brand that does not contain carrageen which is an unhealthy chemical additive. You might also want to experiment with coconut milk, soy milk, cashew milk, or another dairy free option.

Peanut Butter. I use almond butter in any recipe that calls for peanut butter. Read the label to make sure you purchase a brand that has not been processed on equipment that also processes peanuts. Soy butter and sun butter are other alternatives you might want to try.

When my extended family comes for a visit, I make sure that I have a lot of different kinds of fresh fruits and vegetables on hand so that there are healthy nutrient rich foods available for meals and snacks. I keep a bowl of fruit on the counter. I cook a lot of homemade soups and stews. Vic prepare lean meat, chicken, and vegetables on the grill. This allows us to have lots of choices so the folks with food allergies have safe options.

I don't make sweet treats for snacks or waffles for breakfast on a routine basis but I enjoy preparing them when my family comes to visit. Here are recipes for an allergy friendly version of each of these special occasion foods.

Buckeye Balls

This is another holiday treat that is a tradition in my family. However, the original recipe used several processed foods that had chemicals I wanted to avoid and included ingredients that some members of my family cannot consume due to food allergies. I modified the recipe and kept the tradition. Note: If you don't have any food allergies or food sensitivities to contend with you can use milk, real butter, etc. where I've listed alternatives to meet the needs of my allergy crowd.

In a large bowl mix:

1 box of 10 x confectioner sugar

1 ½ cups of almond butter

½ cup of organic non-soy butter substitute

½ cup of organic nonhydrogenated coconut oil

1 teaspoon of pure vanilla extract

Use an electric mixer to cream all of the ingredients together. Then, use your hands to knead the dough into a smooth ball. Break off pieces of dough a tablespoon at a time and form into small balls. Place the balls on a pan or on a cookie sheet lined with wax paper. Stick a toothpick into each ball. Put the balls into the freezer and leave for 1 hour.

Melt 1 bag of Enjoy Life Mini Chocolate Chips and 2 tablespoons of coconut oil in the top of a double boiler. Keep the chocolate over warm water while you dip the balls. Take the balls of dough out of the freezer. Use the toothpick like a little handle to hold the balls while you dip them in the melted chocolate. Dip only the bottom half of each ball in the chocolate leaving a little circle of dough showing at the top. Put on wax paper until the chocolate sets. Remove the toothpicks. Store in an airtight container. These freeze well if you want to make them ahead of time.

Gluten Free Dairy Free Waffles

Note: If you are not cooking for folks with allergies, use regular buttermilk, butter, whole wheat or unbleached flour, etc. to make these yummy waffles.

2 eggs, separated. Beat whites until stiff and set aside.

1 cup of "buttermilk." This is a good technique to use anytime a recipe calls for buttermilk and you need to avoid dairy. Put 1 tablespoon of white vinegar or apple cider vinegar in the bottom of a measuring cup and fill to the 1 cup mark with almond milk or another nondairy milk. Let this mixture sit for at least five minutes.

¼ cup of olive oil

Put 1 tablespoon of almond flour and 1 tablespoon of sorghum flour in a 1 cup measuring cup. Fill the rest of the cup with white rice flour to make 1 cup.

½ cup tapioca flour

1 ½ teaspoon baking soda

1 teaspoon baking powder

Mix dry ingredients in one bowl. In another bowl mix the egg yolks, oil, and milk.

Mix the dry ingredients with the wet ingredients. Then fold in the stiffly beaten egg whites.

Brush a waffle iron with olive oil and preheat.

Bake the waffles on the greased preheated waffle iron.

This recipe makes four large waffles. I use a Belgian waffle maker that creates a round waffle sectioned into four triangles. One of the triangles is enough for one serving for the grandchildren.

For a convenient quick breakfast later, cool the waffles. Cut each waffle into four triangles. Put into a freezer safe container or freezer bag with pieces of waxed paper between each piece. Freeze until ready for use. Defrost and heat in the toaster, a toaster oven, or a regular oven when you want a quick breakfast.

Need more ideas? If you have access to the internet, you have access to an endless supply of healthy recipes. Put a key ingredient plus the word *healthy* in your search engine and dozens of options will pop up on your computer screen. Search Pinterest for healthy eating boards. Follow people on Twitter who tweet organic food recipes. Look for cookbooks that feature organic recipes. Join a Facebook group or page that promotes healthy eating, organic foods, or shares whole food recipes.

Appendix III Resources for Further Reading

Internet links posted were viable links at the time of publication. Internet addresses and product information are offered as a resource and are not intended in any way to be or to imply an endorsement by the authors, Kathy K. Norman or Victor D. Norman. Nor do the authors vouch for the existence, content, or services of these sites beyond the use as resources for the reader.

Websites, Apps, and Social Media Resources
Of course, obviously, I want you to be a part of my social media community. Here are my links.

Website: https://www.kathyknorman.com/
Facebook page: www.facebook.com/practicalpriorities
Pinterest: www.pinterest.com/KathyKNorman3
Twitter: https://twitter.com/kathyknorman

There are many websites, smartphone apps, and social media groups that focus on coping with chronic illness, faith, fibromyalgia, creating a chemical-free life, eating real food, and a wide range of healthy living topics.

Do you love scrolling through Facebook? Join a group or like a page that focuses on chemical-free living, chronic illness, or coping with fibromyalgia.

Hooked on Pinterest? Search for boards to follow that focus on fibromyalgia, healthy living, healthy recipes, and organic cleaners. Addicted to Twitter? Look for the hashtags #healthyliving, #faith, #fibromyalgia, and #HealthyRecipes.

Want to be encouraged? Interested in growing your faith? Follow your favorite spiritual thinkers, writers, and bloggers on your favorite social media platforms.

There are millions of apps and online resources. Here are just a few to give you an idea of what's available.

Apps

There are lots of smartphone apps for checking the ingredients in food, tracking chemical additives in cleaners and cosmetics, and finding the healthiest foods available. Here are a few to get you started. Some of these apps are free. Others charge a small fee.

CosmEthics
Detox Me
EWG's Healthy Living
Fooducate
Non-GMO Project Shopping Guide
Sift Food Labels
Think Dirty – Shop Clean

Websites

Here are a few suggestions from across the web to give you a glimpse of the many possibilities for healthy living websites you can find online.

Centers for Disease Control and Prevention http://www.cdc.gov

Chemical Cuisine https://cspinet.org/eating-healthy/chemical-cuisine

Cleveland Clinic https://my.clevelandclinic.org/health/diseases

Johns Hopkins Medicine https://www.hopkinsmedicine.org/

Mayo Clinic http://www.mayoclinic.org

Medline Plus https://www.nlm.nih.gov/medlineplus

MyFibroTeam https://www.myfibroteam.com
Skin Deep Database http://www.ewg.org/skindeep
Tai Chi for Beginners https://www.youtube.com/watch?v=PNtWqDxwwMg

Twitter
Many of the groups and individuals listed for Twitter can also be found on Facebook, Instagram, Pinterest and other social media platforms. They include real food advocates, faith writers, and fibromyalgia bloggers. Here are ten options from Twitter to give you an idea about what's out there.

@100daysrealfood
@AnnVoskamp
@BethMooreLPM
@eatLocalGrown
@FibroBloggers
@JenHatmaker
@MyFibroTeam
@sarahbessey
@SueInge
@Unbrokensmile1

I appreciate social media and my access to online data. But I also love books. There are lots of great books that are excellent resources for becoming more informed about fibromyalgia, real food, and healthy living. Some of these titles have been on my bookshelf for years, are still well-loved, and often reread. I discovered many of them while completing my personal research project and others in the years since then as I continue to look for ways to eat well, eliminate chemical contamination, and stay healthy. While I don't agree with every single thing in every book, I gained nuggets of useful information from each of them.

Books About Fibromyalgia, Food, and Healthy Living.

100 Days of Real Food: How We Did It, What We Learned, and 100 Easy, Wholesome Recipes Your Family Will Love by Lisa Leake

Animal, Vegetable, Miracle: A Year of Food Life by Barbara Kingsolver

Beat Autoimmune: The Six Keys to Reverse Your Condition and Reclaim Your Health by Palmer Kippola

The Bread Lover's Bread Machine Cookbook by Beth Hensperger

Clean Cuisine: An 8-Week Anti-Inflammatory Diet That Will Change the Way You Age, Look, & Feel by Ivy Ingram Larson and Andrew Larson

Create a Toxin-Free Body & Home Starting Today by W. Lee Cowden, M.D.

The Daniel Plan: 40 Days to a Healthier Life by Rick Warren, Daniel Amen, M.D., and Mark Hyman, M.D.

In Defense of Food: An Eater's Manifesto by Michael Pollan

Eating on the Wild Side: The Missing Link to Optimum Health by Jo Robinson

Eating Well for Optimum Health: The Essential Guide to Bringing Health and Pleasure Back to Eating by Andrew Weil, M. D.

Exercises for Fibromyalgia: The Complete Exercise Guide for Managing and Lessening Fibromyalgia Symptoms by William Smith and Zinovy Meyler

Fast Food Nation: The Dark Side of the All-American Meal by Eric Schlosser

FibroWHYalgia: Why Rebuilding the Ten Root Causes of Chronic Illness Restores Chronic Wellness by Susan E. Ingebretson

Gluten-Free Baking Classics for the Bread Machine by Annalise G. Roberts

The Joy of Cooking by Irma S. Rombauer, Marion Rombauer Becker, and Ethan Becker

Lubkin's Chronic Illness: Impact and Intervention by Pamala D. Larsen

The Maker's Diet: The 40-Day Health Experience That Will Change Your Life Forever by Jordan S. Rubin

Mayo Clinic Guide to Fibromyalgia: Strategies to Take Back Your Life by Andy Abril, M.D and Barbara Kay Bruce, Ph.D.

More-With-Less Cookbook by Doris Janzen Longacre

New Hope for People with Fibromyalgia by Theresa Foy DiGeronimo

Salt Sugar Fat: How the Food Giants Hooked Us by Michael Moss

Super Immunity: The Essential Nutrition Guide for Boosting Your Body's Defenses by Joel Fuhrman, M.D.

This Is How I Save My Life: From California to India, a True Story Of Finding Everything When You Are Willing To Try Anything by Amy B. Scher

The Whole30: The 30-Day Guide to Total Health and Food Freedom by Melissa Hartwig Urban

Books About Faith and Spirituality

It encourages me to read books written by a diverse group of people from different cultural backgrounds and faith traditions that have wide ranging theological perspectives. Some of these suggestions are well-loved and dogeared books I've owned for years. Others are recent discoveries. I have been enlightened and informed by reading books written by mainline Christians, Jewish rabbis, Protestant women, Catholic priests, liberal thinkers, and unaffiliated spiritual seekers. Here are a few suggestions for readers interested in spirituality and faith.

1000 Gifts: A Dare to Live Fully Right Where You Are by Ann Voskamp

An Altar in the World: A Geography of Faith by Barbara Brown Taylor

Candles in the Dark: Letters of Hope and Encouragement by Amy Carmichael

Celebration of Discipline: The Path to Spiritual Growth by Richard J. Foster

For the Love: Fighting for Grace in a World of Impossible Standards by Jen Hatmaker

Help, Thanks, Wow: The Three Essential Prayers by Anne Lamott

The Hiding Place by Corrie Ten Boom

Inspired: Slaying Giants, Walking on Water, and Loving the Bible Again by Rachel Held Evans

Learning to Pray When Your Heart is Breaking by Denise George

Letters and Papers from Prison by Dietrich Bonhoeffer

Mere Christianity by C.S. Lewis

Of Mess and Moxie: Wrangling Delight Out of This Wild and Glorious Life by Jen Hatmaker

Miracles and Other Reasonable Things: A Story of Unlearning and Relearning God by Sarah Bessey

Out of Sorts: Making Sense of an Evolving Faith by Sarah Bessey

A Place of Healing: Wrestling with the Mysteries of Suffering by Joni Eareckson Tada

Prayer: Does It Make Any Difference? By Philip Yancey

The Ragamuffin Gospel: Good News for the Bedraggled, Beat-Up, and Burnt Out by Brennan Manning

Searching for Sunday: Loving, Leaving, and Finding the Church by Rachel Held Evans

A Shepherd Looks at Psalm 23 by Phillip Keller

Simplicity: The Freedom of Letting Go by Richard Rohr

Small Victories: Spotting Improbable Moments of Grace by Anne Lamott

Tracks of a Fellow Struggler: Living and Growing Through Grief by John Claypool

When Bad Things Happen to Good People by Harold S. Kushner

When Your Rope Breaks by Steve Brown

Acknowledgments

Creating this book has been a long journey of small steps that occurred at just the right time to push me finally to write everything down. I'm grateful to all my friends and family, fellow fibromyalgia sufferers, physicians, pastors, my social media community, random acquaintances, and anyone and everyone who gave me encouragement, information, and motivation to keep writing. I appreciate each of you. I want to take this opportunity to thank a few of you by name. Thanks to Donna Hanby Pridmore for sharing the article she saw in the newspaper about an upcoming Boot Camp for Christian Writers Conference at Samford University and for encouraging me to attend. Boot Camp gave me the kick-start I needed. Thank you to author Denise George, founder of Writers for Life, for exceptional seminars and encouragement at every Boot Camp workshop, and for the enthusiastic endorsement of this book. Thanks to Susan Hord Herman, at Rhuby Editorial, for the wise developmental editing when I had only a handful of pages and a tiny germ of an idea. Thanks to Holly N. McKinney, editor extraordinaire, for the outstanding final copy edit of the manuscript. Thank you to Luke Norman for being my personal IT consultant. I never would have survived all the technological hurdles without his wisdom and assistance. Thanks to Dr. Chris George, senior pastor of Smoke Rise Baptist Church, for allowing me to use his sermon, "Hot, Humid, and Hungry" in telling my story. Thank you to Kay M. Williams, for agreeing to be my beta reader, for trying the strategies for recovery, and for the lovely endorsement of their validity. Thank you to Dr. William H. Coleman, M.D. and Dr. M. Dennis Herman, D. Min. for taking the time to read the manuscript and endorse the book. Thank you to Cheryl Sloan Wray and all the fine folks at the Southern Christian Writers Conference for every workshop, resource, and word of encouragement. A special thanks to Cheryl and SCWC Books for publishing the eBook for Practical Priorities for Fibromyalgia Recovery. Thank you to Alice Briggs at Kingdom Covers for assistance with formatting and cover design for the print version of the book. And forever and always, thank you to my husband, Vic Norman, who surprised me with the gift of my first tiny green screened computer almost 40 years ago when I said I wanted to be a writer, encouraged me as I published articles in Christian magazines way back then, and supported me in countless ways, when after quite a long hiatus. I said I wanted to start writing again. I am so grateful that when I asked him to contribute to this book by sharing his medical expertise, he said, "Yes."

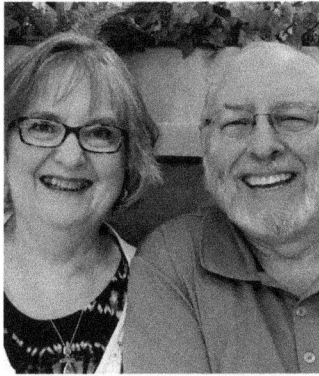

About the Authors

Kathy K. Norman is a previously published author of devotionals, Bible studies, and lifestyle pieces for Christian magazines. She is an educator, blogger, and healthy living advocate. Kathy is familiar with the medical world from working in her husband's clinic.

After numerous requests to share the strategies she created to cope with the severe symptoms of fibromyalgia syndrome, Kathy wrote Practical Priorities for Fibromyalgia Recovery in conjunction with her husband, Victor D. Norman, M.D., a board-certified family physician and medical educator. Dr. Norman graduated from the University of Alabama School of Medicine, was a family physician for thirty years, and was a member of the faculty of the University of Alabama School of Medicine, Huntsville Campus.

The Normans served together as missionaries in Barranquilla, Colombia, South America. Practical Priorities for Fibromyalgia Recovery is their first book collaboration. They love to travel and camp in their motorhome. So far, they have checked the Grand Canyon, Yellowstone and Glacier National Parks, the Painted Desert, the Petrified Forest, and the Canadian Rockies off their camping bucket list.

Visit Kathy's website for updates on her current writing projects and adventures.

https://www.kathyknorman.com/

Endnotes

1 "Fibromyalgia Prevalence." National Fibromyalgia Association. https://fmaware.net/fibromyalgia-prevalence/ (1997-2020) Web. June 1, 2020.

2 "What Are the Signs and Symptoms of Fibromyalgia?" Centers for Disease Control and Prevention. https://www.cdc.gov/arthritis/basics/fibromyalgia.htm (11 October, 2017) Web. June 1, 2020.

3 "Chronic Illness and Depression". Cleveland Clinic. https://my.clevelandclinic.org/health/articles/9288-chronic-illness-and-depression (17 January, 2017) Web. June 1, 2020.

4 Younger, Jarred. "Fibromyalgia Best Treated as an Inflammatory Disease." Helio Rheumatology. Congress of Clinical Rheumatology Annual Meeting. https://www.healio.com/news/rheumatology/20180525/fibromyalgia-best-treated-as-inflammatory-disease (29 May, 2018) Web. June 3, 2020.

5 Azab, Marwa, PhD. "The Brain on Fire: Depression and Inflammation." Psychology Today. https://www.psychologytoday.com/us/blog/neuroscience-in-everyday-life/201810/the-brain-fire-depression-and-inflammation (29 October, 2018) Web. June 1, 2020.

6 Bell, J.R., C.M. Baldwin, and G.E. Schwartz. "Illness from Low Levels of Environmental Chemicals: Relevance to Chronic Fatigue Syndrome and Fibromyalgia." National Institutes

of Health. National Center for Biotechnology Information. https://pubmed.ncbi.nlm.nih.gov/9790486/ (28 September, 1998) Web. June 3, 2020.

7   "Household Chemical Products and Their Health Risk." Cleveland Clinic. https://my.clevelandclinic.org/health/article s/11397-household-chemical-products-and-their-health-risk (24 May, 2018) Web. June 3, 2020.

8   "50 Jawdroppingly Toxic Food Ingredients & Artificial Additives to Avoid." Masters of Public Health Programs List. https://mphprogramslist.com/50-jawdroppingly-toxic-foo d-additives-to-avoid/ (2020 MPHProgramsList) Web. June 3, 2020

9   "Almost a quarter of all disease caused by environmental exposure." World Health Organization. https://www.who. int/mediacentre/news/releases/2006/pr32/en/ (16 June, 2006) Web. June 3, 2020

10 Sears, Margaret E., and Stephen J. Genuis. "Environmental Determinants of Chronic Disease and Medical Approaches: Recognition, Avoidance, Supportive Therapy, and Detoxification." Hindawi. Journal of Environmental and Public Health. https://www.hindawi.com/journals/ jeph/2012/356798/ (19 January, 2012) Web. June 3, 2020.

11 "Is Food Coloring Safe for Kids?" Cleveland Clinic. Health Essentials. https://health.clevelandclinic.org/is-foo d-coloring-safe-for-kids/ (26 December, 2019) Web. June 8, 2020. Kobylewski, Sarah and Michael F. Jacobson. "Toxicology of Food Dyes." National Institutes of Health. National Library of Medicine. https://pubmed.ncbi.nlm. nih.gov/23026007/ (July 2012) Web. June 8, 2020.

12 Mawer, Rudy. "6 Reasons Why High Fructose Corn Syrup is Bad for You." Healthline. https://www.healthline.com/nutri-tion/why-high-fructose-corn-syrup-is-bad#1 (27 September, 2019) Web. June 8, 2020.

13 Gunners, Kris. "Are Nitrates and Nitrites in Food Harmful?" Healthline. https://www.healthline.com/

nutrition/are-nitrates-and-nitrites-harmful (10 February, 2020) Web. June 8, 2020. Ma, Linsha and Liang Hu, et al. "Nitrate and Nitrite in Health and Disease." National Center for Biotechnology Information. U.S. Library of Aging and Medicine. https://www.ncbi.nlm.nih.gov/pmc/articles/PMC6147587/ (1 October, 2018) Web. June 8, 2020.

14 "Formaldehyde." American Cancer Society. https://www.cancer.org/cancer/cancer-causes/formaldehyde.html (23 May, 2014) Web. June 8, 2020.

15 "BPA and Phthalates." Westchester County Department of Health. https://health.westchestergov.com/bisphenol-a-and-phthalates#:~:text=It%20is%20believed%20that%20both,including%20hormonal%20and%20devel-opmental%20problems. (2020) Web. June 8, 2020. Singh, Sher and Steven Shoei-Lung Li. "Epigenetic Effects of Environmental Chemicals Bisphenol A and Phthalates." International Journal of Molecular Sciences. MDPI. https://www.mdpi.com/1422-0067/13/8/10143 (15 August, 2012) June 8, 2020.

16 "BHA and BHT: A Case for Fresh?" Scientific American. https://www.scientificamerican.com/article/bha-and-bht-a-case-for-fresh/ (19 December, 2013) Web. June 8, 2020.

17 "Chemical Pesticides and Human Health: The Urgent Need for a New Concept in Agriculture." Frontiers in Public Health. National Institutes of Health. https://www.ncbi.nlm.nih.gov/pmc/articles/PMC4947579/ (18 July, 2016) Web. June 8, 2020.

18 Potera, Carol. "Indoor Air Quality: Scented Products Emit a Bouquet of VOCs." Environmental Health Perspectives. US National Library of Medicine. National Institutes of Health. https://www.ncbi.nlm.nih.gov/pmc/articles/PMC3018511/ (January, 2011) Web. June 12, 2020.

19 Ferlow, Klaus. "Fragrance: A Growing Health and Environmental Hazard. Part 1." Stason.org. https://stason.

org/articles/wellbeing/health/environment/Fragrance-A-Growing-Health-and-Environmental-Hazard-Part-1.html (2018) Web. June 29, 2020.

20 "Volatile Organic Compounds Impact on Indoor Air Quality." United States Environmental Protection Agency. https://www.epa.gov/indoor-air-quality-iaq/volatile-organic-compounds-impact-indoor-air-quality#:~:text=Health%20effects%20may%20include%3A,kidney%20and%20central%20nervous%20system (19 January, 2017) Web. June 29, 2020.

21 Singla, Veena. "Not Just Dirt: Toxic Chemicals in Indoor Dust." Natural Resources Defense Council. https://www.nrdc.org/resources/not-just-dirt-toxic-chemicals-indoor-dust#:~:text=Toxic%20Chemicals%20in%20Dust%20%3D%20Public%20Health%20Threats&text=Some%20phthalates%2C%20fragrance%2C%20flame%20retardants,10%20chemicals%20found%20in%20dust. (14 September, 2016) Web. June 29, 2020.

22 Burns, Carla. "Natural or Organic Cosmetics? Don't Trust Marketing Claims." Environmental Working Group. https://www.ewg.org/news-and-analysis/2018/01/natural-or-organic-cosmetics-don-t-trust-marketing-claims (11 January, 2018) Web. June 29, 2020.

23 McCullough, Donna M. "Environmental Diseases from A to Z." National Institute of Health. National Institute of Environmental Health Sciences." https://www.niehs.nih.gov/health/assets/docs_a_e/environmental_diseases_environmental_diseases_from_a_to_z_english_508.pdf (June 2007) Web. June 29, 2020.

24 Smith, Amy and Amy Richter, RD. "How Do Processed Foods Affect Your Health?" Medical News Today. https://www.medicalnewstoday.com/articles/318630 (14 May, 2020) Web. July 10, 2020.

25 Shelton, Richard C., M.D. and Andrew H. Miller, M.D. "Inflammation in Depression: Is Adiposity a Cause?" Dialogues in Clinical Neuroscience. National Institutes of Health. (13 March, 2011) Web. July 10, 2020.

26 Benzaken, Hilla. "5 Super Simple Ways to Get Pesticides Off Your Produce." Goodnet. https://www.goodnet.org/articles/5-super-simple-ways-to-get-pesticides-off-your-produce (17 October, 2018) Web. July 15, 2020.

27 Villines, Zawn and Gregory Minnis, DPT. "Best Exercises for Fibromyalgia." Medical News Today. https://www.medicalnewstoday.com/articles/321506 (16 April, 2018) Web. July 15, 2020.

28 Suzuki, Katsuhiko. "Cytokine Response to Exercise and Its Modulation." Antioxidants. MDPI. US National Library of Medicine. https://www.ncbi.nlm.nih.gov/pmc/articles/PMC5789327/ (17 January, 2018) Web. July 15, 2020.

Internet links posted in the endnotes were viable links at the time of publication. Any internet addresses or company or product information printed in this book are offered as a resource and are not intended in any way to be or to imply an indorsement by the authors, Kathy K. Norman or Victor D. Norman. Nor do the authors vouch for the existence, content, or services of these sites beyond the use as resources for the reader.

www.ingramcontent.com/pod-product-compliance
Lightning Source LLC
Chambersburg PA
CBHW032131020426
42334CB00016B/1119